Samia ABBASSENE
Boualem SEMAOUNE

Burnout among general practitioners in Algeria

Samia ABBASSENE
Boualem SEMAOUNE

Burnout among general practitioners in Algeria

Descriptive study of the syndrome among general practitioners in the Wilaya of Setif

ScienciaScripts

Imprint
Any brand names and product names mentioned in this book are subject to trademark, brand or patent protection and are trademarks or registered trademarks of their respective holders. The use of brand names, product names, common names, trade names, product descriptions etc. even without a particular marking in this work is in no way to be construed to mean that such names may be regarded as unrestricted in respect of trademark and brand protection legislation and could thus be used by anyone.

Cover image: www.ingimage.com

This book is a translation from the original published under ISBN 978-620-6-73564-9.

Publisher:
Sciencia Scripts
is a trademark of
Dodo Books Indian Ocean Ltd. and OmniScriptum S.R.L publishing group

120 High Road, East Finchley, London, N2 9ED, United Kingdom
Str. Armeneasca 28/1, office 1, Chisinau MD-2012, Republic of Moldova, Europe
Managing Directors: Ieva Konstantinova, Victoria Ursu
info@omniscriptum.com

Printed at: see last page
ISBN: 978-620-4-18961-1

Contents

"Medicine is a disease that strikes all doctors unequally. Some reap lasting benefits.

Others decide one day to hand in their smocks, because it's the only way to heal, at the cost of a few scars.

Whether we like it or not, we are still doctors. But you don't have to make other people pay for it, and you don't have to die for it either"[i].

ACKNOWLEDGEMENTS

To Professor SEMAOUNE Bouaíem
Thank you' for agreeing to supervise this thesis
For being so present and supportive despite the distance
For accompanying me throughout this tedious work
Thank you for your availability, even at weekends and on public holidays.
Thank you for listening and for your invaluable help.
It's an honour and a pleasure to work with you.
Please accept my sincere gratitude.

To Professor BENCHARF Mohamed El Amin.
You do me the honour of chairing my jury
Please accept' the expression of my deepest respect
Please accept my sincerest thanks.

To Professor BAGHDADLI Benati
Thank you' for agreeing to be one of' the members of my jury
Please accept my warmest thanks

To Professor HAMADOUCHE Mohamed
I am pleased to count you among the members of my jury.
Thank you for your encouragement, support and help
Please find herewith the expression of my consideration and gratitude

To Professor KHOUDOUR Zoubida
You have agreed to sit on my jury
Please accept' the expression of my deepest respect

To Professor LAOUAMRISUmane
For your cooperation and help.

To Professor DJABI Farda
For your support, your availability and your kindness

To Mr SANA Mourad *of the DSP for having facilitated my access to the various establishments to carry out this work.*

To the YAHIA FAMiLY*: for their undeniable family spirit*

To my friends Amira, ***Ouahba and Hafdha*** *for their sincere friendship. You are always there at the right time.*

To my long-time friends ***Rebha K, Samba A and Ouahba R.***

To my colleagues and friends in the department: ***Dr RAHMANI Nassima*** *and* ***Dr BOUKRAA Aissa*** *For their presence and encouragement*

To the work doctors ***BELAMRI AND*** *AKMOUM* ***for*** *their ongoing help and support. Thank you and stay yourself*

To my colleagues and friends ***CHAKER SLASLEDJ W, MOHAMMEDIH, ZEGHAD K HASS AD S, KOUACHI A, REGGAD M, TOUATI A, TOUABT A ET BOUAKAZ M.***
Thank you for your help

To the staff of *the occupational medicine department who, in one way or another have*

accompanied and supported me throughout my working life.
To Dr HABBECHE Samir *from Béni Ourtiène for his extreme kindness.*
To Mr BENMAIZIA A *of Mostaganem, for his invaluable help in the field of biostatistics.*
To all the ***general practitioners*** *who took the time to reply to the questionnaire*

INTRODUCTION

In the world of work, the importance of finance and economics is increasing to the detriment of the quality of human relations, and more and more workers are suffering morally.
After a long university career, doctors are expected to be competent, available and unfailingly responsible for the demands of the medical profession. In the eyes of society, the doctor is at the service of the patient.
It's a demanding discipline whose mission requires a great deal of commitment and sacrifice. The already high level of investment seems to be growing in tandem with the constraints. However, faced with the multiple constraints of medical responsibility, work overload, lack of resources, aggressive patient behaviour and the directing and intransigent attitude of the administration, doctors find themselves in great distress.
Burnout, the term used to describe this state of extreme suffering, has an impact not only on the physical and psychological health of doctors, but also on the quality of the care they provide.
It is being studied more and more [2-8], and the various studies carried out in different countries confirm its existence in this socio-professional category. For a long time, burnout was a taboo subject, since in society's eyes the doctor was the carer, not the patient. As a result, carers are often the first to deny that they suffer from burnout, even though it is a reality that has been proven by numerous studies.
In Algeria, it has to be admitted that very few studies have been published on the subject [9-14]; and given the unease that we also felt among our doctors, the idea of a study was obvious to us.
We therefore thought it would be interesting to carry out this study among general practitioners in the wilaya of Sétif in order to assess the prevalence rate of burnout syndrome in this population and to estimate its 3 dimensions, namely emotional exhaustion (EE), depersonalisation (DP) and personal accomplishment (PA).
We will determine the factors that predispose to burnout and identify its consequences.
Finally, proposals for preventive action will be put forward.
We hope that this study will contribute to a better understanding of the factors involved in physician burnout, in the hope of improving the means of countering it.

THEORETICAL PART

1. THEORETICAL BACKGROUND

1.1 HISTORY

It is important to detail the origins and development of burnout (Burn Out, BO) to explain the difficulty of its acceptance by the scientific community[15].

This is not a new syndrome [16], as it has been used before, under different names:

Intellectual overwork by Desoille and Raynaud, managerial overwork by Bize and Goguelin[15], industrial fatigue by Myers in 1921[16], neurosis of telephone operators and mechanographers by Le Guillant and Bégoin[16, 17 , 18], states of exhaustion in 1959 by psychiatrist Claude Veil[15].

Etymologically speaking, the term "exhaustion" refers to the fact of "emptying the water from a well when too much has already been removed". According to Lebigot & Lafont [19], the term therefore has a metaphorical value. In France, this term is used instead.

As for the term burnout, historians trace its origins back to 1969 [16], but according to Schaufeli and Enzmann it is not a new phenomenon: "It has its roots in the past" [20].

The verb 'to burn out' was used by Shakespeare in 1599 [16, 20] and, according to Kleiber and Enzmann, the word was incorporated into the English vocabulary in 1900 to designate excessive work leading to early death [16].

In 1969, the term was first used in psychology by H.B. Bradley in an article describing a particular kind of work-related stress[21].

Although Bradley was the first to use the term [22], it is the American Herbert J Freudenberger who is generally considered to be the spiritual father of the burnout syndrome [23], since it was he who initiated the first theoretical reflections on the subject [16].

In 1974, he published an article entitled Staff Burn-Out in the Journal of Social Issues.

Herbert J. Freudenberger is a psychiatrist and psychoanalyst practising in New York at a free clinic for drug addicts.

Free clinics are private, not-for-profit therapeutic centres that operate mainly with young volunteers, who must be available to treat this category of patient.

He uses this term to describe a condition that he and other volunteers develop after a year. These initially enthusiastic carers lose their dynamism, commitment and motivation and present physical symptoms (feelings of exhaustion and fatigue, headaches, gastro-intestinal problems, various somatic complaints, insomnia, etc.) and behavioural symptoms (presence of a series of signs such as frustration, irritability, anger, crying, etc.).) and behavioural symptoms (signs such as frustration, irritability, anger, crying, negative and cynical attitudes towards patients, inability to cope with new situations, loss of energy).

There is alcohol or psychotropic drug abuse and the person acts as if depressed. They work hard and spend a lot of time at work, but are ineffective.

He uses the term with reference to the dictionary definition: the verb "to burn out" means "to fail, wear out or become exhausted as a result of an excessive demand on one's energy, strength or resources"[24], and is also a metaphor for the effect of chronic drug use[22, 25, 26].

Justifying this metaphorical term, Freudenberger said later in 1980: *"I realised in the course of my daily practice that people are sometimes victims of fire just like buildings; under the strain produced by our complex world, their internal resources come to be consumed as if by flames, leaving nothing but an immense void inside, even if the external envelope seems more or less intact*"[15].

Freudenberger and Richelson believe that burnout mainly affects people who overestimate themselves, seeing themselves as dynamic, charismatic and competent[27].

At the same time, around 1976, Christina Maslach, a researcher in social psychology, was interested in the strategies developed by health and social services staff to cope with the high emotional demands of their profession.

As the term burnout is familiar to Californian lawyers working with people in social difficulty, describing progressive exhaustion, a cynical attitude and a loss of commitment, she decided to adopt it for her research[22, 23].

Even though burnout became very popular as soon as it was introduced, the scientific community received it with great suspicion[15]; Maslach's article for a scientific journal was returned to him on the grounds that it was "pop psychology"[22].

Unlike Freudenberger, who emphasises personal factors, Maslach locates the causes of burnout in the work environment [23].

Clinicians have therefore focused on the symptoms of burnout and mental health problems, while psychologists have looked at the relationship between carer and cared-for and the professional context [20, 26].

Most early research was descriptive and qualitative, using techniques such as interviews, case studies and observation [26, 28].

In the early 1980s, empirical research into burnout was carried out methodically, on a large number of subjects and using questionnaires. During this period, a validated measurement instrument with solid psychometric qualities was used: the *Maslach Burn out Inventory (MBI)* developed by Maslach and Jackson in 1981 [20, 22, 26, 29].

In 1980, Cherniss proposed a transactional view, in which burnout is the product of an interaction between an individual and his environment, which are not separate entities but components of an evolving process that continuously influences each other [23, 30].

The imbalance between individual and organisational resources in the face of work demands results in stress, which leads to tension, emotional exhaustion and anxiety [23].

In 1982, Pines proposed a motivational approach to the syndrome. According to her, work represents an existential quest, and burnout develops when there is a gap between work expectations and reality (inability to find existential meaning in one's work)[30, 31].

In the mid-1990s, the concept of burnout was extended to other professional fields, as the characteristics of burnout were identified outside the helping professions[32].

In scientific terms, "burnout" or "burnout syndrome" are still regarded with caution in psychiatric circles and in the field of occupational medicine [15, 30].

1.2 SYMPTOMS AND CONSEQUENCES OF BURNOUT

132 symptoms of burnout have been identified in the form of a primer: from A for anxiety to Z for lack of zeal [33].

Burnout has negative consequences for doctors' health and for the healthcare relationship[34].

As it is often difficult to distinguish between the symptoms and consequences of burnout, it seems preferable to use the term "manifestations" [22].

1.2.1 Manifestations of BO according to certain authors

The manifestations are diverse and are classified from three to seven different aspects depending on the author [35].

KAHILL(1988) proposes a grouping of events into five categories:

physical, emotional, interpersonal, attitudinal and behavioural [29].

1.2.2 BO events selected by Schaufeli and Enzmann

In 1998, Schaufeli and Enzmann identified five categories which are expressed at an individual level, but also at interpersonal and organisational levels: affective, cognitive, physical, behavioural and motivational [33].

According to Burisch (2010), symptoms can be divided into 7 main categories [16].

We will now look in more detail at the five categories of event identified by Schaufeli and Enzmann.

1.2.2.1 Affective

The person is emotionally 'drained' and has a depressed mood with a sense of failure, powerlessness and hopelessness.

She experiences ill-defined fears and anxiety, and is frequently irritable and quick to anger or cry.

1.2.2.2 Cognitive

Impaired memory, attention and concentration, with difficulty in making decisions. Low self-esteem and suicidal ideation.

1.2.2.3 Physics

All kinds of non-specific complaints can be seen, such as headaches, nausea, eating disorders, digestive problems, musculoskeletal pain and sleep disorders.

However, the most typical physical manifestation of BO is a feeling of chronic fatigue.

People suffering from BO may experience prolonged or recurrent infections as a result of reduced immune defences. Cardiovascular problems have also been described.

1.2.2.4 Behavioural

Abandonment of social and leisure activities, with the possibility of addictive behaviour: tobacco, alcohol, coffee, drugs and tranquillisers.

In the workplace, hyperactivity and restlessness may be seen, while being less and less effective (presenteeism), and procrastination, doubts and indecision may be observed.

1.2.2.5 Motivational

Decreased motivation for work, manifested by reduced commitment, loss of interest and idealism.

The subject is discouraged, disappointed, takes no initiative and lacks zeal.

1.3 TERMS USED

Three different expressions are currently used to describe this syndrome.

1.3.1 Burnout syndrome

When **Freudenberger** used this original expression in his 1974 article, he referred to the dictionary definition.

The verb "to burn-out" means "to fail, wear out or become exhausted as a result of an excessive demand on one's energy, strength or resources".

The term burnout describes the state of a candle which, after lighting for long hours, offers only a discreet and weak flame [36].

It refers to total combustion, the reduction to ashes of a completely burnt-out object from which all the matter has disappeared.

In the aerospace industry, the image is more evocative: depletion of a rocket's fuel, resulting in overheating and machine breakdown [15, 25].

1.3.2 Karoshi or Karôshi

Pronounced Kaloshi. Japanese term for "death from overwork".

In a culture governed by the notion of the collective good, employees sacrifice themselves to satisfy the demands of others and their company. They give countless hours of their time and work themselves to exhaustion. To live and die for the company could be the Japanese precept, so prevalent is the desire for success and excellence[15]. The first case of death was reported in 1969[37], which drew attention to the harmful effects of overwork.

Three doctors, Hosokawa, Tajiri and Uehata, gave a detailed description of this syndrome, which they called "Karoshi" (®^^, death by labour) [38].

It occurs in young men, managers or employees aged between twenty-five and forty, with no history of cardiovascular disease, following a cerebral haemorrhage or myocardial infarction. In Japan, *karôshi* been recognised as an occupational disease since the 1970s [17].

1.3.3 Burnout syndrome

This term is vague and seems to encompass all the effects of work on the individual. It is a pale reflection of the more colourful term burnout.

Usure professionnelle or usure au travail are also expressions used. However, despite all these criticisms, it is this term that has come to dominate the French language[15].

1.4 DEFINITIONS

A large number of researchers have taken an interest in this issue, generating a plethora of definitions.

Indeed, the first major review of the literature published in 1982 listed no fewer than 48 definitions in articles published between 1974 and 1980 [39], which is one of the major obstacles to research into burnout.

We quote the following definitions:

In 1974, Herbert J. Freudenberger proposed an initial definition which D. Bérard and A. Duquette give the following translation:

"Burnout is a condition caused by the excessive use of one's energy and resources, resulting in a feeling of failure, exhaustion or burnout"[15].

With Richelson in 1980, he describes it as "a state of fatigue or frustration caused by devotion to a cause, lifestyle or relationship that fails to produce the desired results"[27].

Maslach and his colleagues have proposed the following definitions:

In 1976 as "an inability of the worker to adapt to a continuous level of emotional stress caused by the work environment"[15].

"A syndrome of emotional exhaustion, depersonalisation and reduced personal fulfilment that appears in individuals who are professionally involved with others" [28, 40], this definition has become the benchmark for research in the field [41].

"It represents an erosion of values, dignity, spirit and will - an erosion of the human soul. It represents an erosion of values, dignity, spirit and will - an erosion of the human soul. It's a suffering that builds progressively and continuously, sucking the subject into a downward spiral from which it's difficult to extricate oneself... Three things happen: you feel chronically exhausted; you become cynical and detached from your work; and you feel increasingly ineffective in your job"[42].

"A syndrome that develops following prolonged exposure to work-related emotional and interpersonal stressors, and is characterised by the three dimensions of exhaustion, cynicism and inefficiency"[26].

For Cherniss (1980), it is "a process in which a previously involved employee withdraws in reaction to the demands and burdens of his or her job" [16].

Edelwich and Brodsky (1980) describe "a gradual decline in idealism, energy, ambition and participation as a result of working conditions" [16].

For Pines and Aronson in 1988, it is defined as "a state of physical, emotional and mental exhaustion caused by long-term involvement in emotionally demanding situations". According to Pines, these demanding situations are not only found at work [37].

It is therefore a shifting concept with multiple definitions, none of which can claim to synthesise it[43].

These definitions complement rather than oppose each other. They reveal the complexity of burnout, which can in fact be explained by several models and result from many interrelated causes[37].

1.5 DESCRIPTION OF THE SYNDROME

Maslach provided a better understanding of burnout by describing it as a three-dimensional phenomenon. The three fundamental dimensions of this syndrome have not only opened up prospects for assessment, but also for psychodynamic understanding and therapeutic approaches [15].

The 3 fundamental dimensions of the syndrome :

- Emotional exhaustion (EE)
- Depersonalisation (DP) or dehumanisation of the relationship with others
- Reduced personal fulfilment (PA)

1.5.1 EMOTIONAL EXHAUSTION (EE)

Emotional exhaustion is as much physical as psychological [42], and most authors consider it to be the key component of the syndrome.

This is a state of tiredness that results in an almost total absence of emotional energy, which will have repercussions on the individual's physical vitality.

This unusual fatigue is significant and is not improved by rest, and the thought of having to face another day seems insurmountable to the individual[44].

Externally, there may be emotional outbursts such as crying spells or fits of temper, as well as a refusal to act or to respond to even innocuous requests[15].

The emotionally exhausted individual is no longer capable of helping others.

This component represents the stress dimension of burnout [26, 45].

1.5.2 DEPERSONALISATION OR DEHUMANISATION OF THE RELATIONSHIP WITH OTHERS (DP)

Depersonalisation or dehumanisation of the relationship with others represents the second dimension of OO. It is ***the hard core of*** the syndrome [15].

This is a negative, detached, even cynical attitude on the part of the individual towards the people with whom they interact in their professional context (patients, colleagues or clients), who end up being treated like objects, leading to cold and distant relationships [35], with a loss of empathy [17].

This excessive detachment is often accompanied by a loss of idealism [45]. This state develops gradually and slowly. Distancing oneself from the other is often painfully experienced as a form of personal failure, but this attitude is seen as an adaptation and protection strategy that enables the person to continue to work on their relationships [15].

This component represents the interpersonal dimension of the burnout phenomenon[45].

In the medical field, the patient is no longer considered as a person but rather as an object: a case or a room number[15].the doctor looks after the diseased organ, disregarding the personality of his patient, whom he describes with cynicism and omnipotence[46].

According to Canoui, the term "depersonalization" used by Maslach and Jackson in French psychiatric semiology refers to a disorder of consciousness during which the subject experiences the impression of the transformation of his personality and the modification of his body. The term should therefore not be retained in French, since burnout involves a change in the relationship with others, a loss of empathy and a difficulty in recognising the person in others. For this reason, he believes that the term "dehumanisation of the interpersonal relationship" would be more appropriate [15]. However, even in the English language, according to Schaufeli, the term can lead to some confusion: in psychiatry, it is used to refer to a person's extreme alienation from themselves and the world, whereas in Maslach and Jackson's definition, it refers to an impersonal and dehumanised perception of others, rather than an impersonal vision of the self[22].

1.5.3 REDUCED PERSONAL ACHIEVEMENT (AP)

This dimension is the consequence of the other two: being emotionally exhausted and no longer interested in others, personal fulfilment declines[47].

This is a feeling of personal ineffectiveness, with the onset of demotivation, guilt, low self-esteem and loss of confidence.

The consequences vary: absenteeism, dropping out of work, lack of rigour or even professional errors and a loss of interest in the job for some.

In others, on the contrary, we observe an over-investment in work called "presenteeism", with the production of totally ineffective work. Loss of self-confidence is associated with major depression[25].

The decrease in the sense of personal accomplishment represents the self-evaluation dimension of burnout[45].

I.6 MEASUREMENT SCALES

With the problem of assessment posed, a large number of scales measuring burnout are being tested.

1.6.1 The different measurement scales

Burnout Questionnaire by Freudenberger and Richelson (1980), Individual Burnout Symptomatic Questionnaire by Appelbaum (1980), Staff Burnout Scale by Jones (1980), Emener-Luck Burnout Scale by Emener, Luck and Gohs (1982), Job Burnout Inventory by Ford, Murphy and Edwards (1983), Meier Burnout Assessment by Meier (1984), EnergyDepletion Index by Garden (1985), Cherniss Burnout Measure by Burke and Deszca (1986), Matthews Burnout Scale for Employees by Matthews (1986), Teacher Burnout Scale by Seidman and Zager (1986-1987), Boudreau Burnout Questionnaire (2006), Bergen Burnout Inventory (2010), Shirom-Melamed Burnout Measure by Shirom and Melamed (2006)[16], TediumMeasure by Pines and Aronson (1981)[48], Oldenburg Burnout Inventory by Demerouti, Bakker, Vardakou&.Kantas (2003)[49], The Copenhagen Burnout Inventory (CBI)[50].

1.6.2 Maslach Burnout Inventory (MBI)

However, the Maslach Burnout Inventory (MBI) developed by Maslach and his team has the most solid psychometric qualities [26] and is therefore by far the most widely used, currently covering around 90% of the literature in this field [16, 51, 52].The translation of Maslach and Jackson's burnout inventory (MBI) into French has been validated by Dion and Tessier and has satisfactory psychometric qualities [48].This scale will enable research to develop rapidly in various countries [53].

1.6.2.1 Presentation of the tool

In 1981, Maslach published the Maslach Burnout Inventory [28].

1.6.2.1.1 Initial version

In its initial version, the tool had four components: criteria for emotional exhaustion, dehumanisation, personal fulfilment and commitment to work, explored by 47 items which were then reduced to 25 and validated using the statistical method of factorial analysis.
These items are assessed using two scales (Likert-type frequency and intensity scale)

- a frequency scale rated from 0 to 6 (from never to every day)
- an intensity scale rated from 1 to 7 (from very little to a great deal)

This version was administered to workers whose professions are known to expose them to burnout: police officers, teachers, nurses, social workers, psychologists, lawyers, doctors, etc. [54].

1.6.2.1.2 Final shape

In its final form, the "commitment to work" component was not retained and the tool presents 22 items exploring the three dimensions:

- emotional exhaustion (9 items)
- dehumanisation (5 items)
- personal fulfilment (8 items)

At present, given the strong correlation observed between the intensity and frequency scales in the various studies, the authors have retained only the frequency scale [15, 40].
This first version of the tool was designed for aid professionals.
As the syndrome was extended to all professions, the use of the MBI did require adaptation, which led Maslach to develop other versions in 1986.
There are currently 3 versions of the MBI [40]:

- The original version: the MBI - HSS (the MBI- Human Services Survey)
- The MBI- ES (MBI-Educators Survey) for education professionals
- the MBI- GS (MBI-General Survey) for other categories of professionals where contact with the public is less central.

It comprises 16 items (5 items for "emotional exhaustion", 5 for depersonalisation which is called "cynicism" and 6 for professional fulfilment which is called "professional effectiveness".
In its three forms, the MBI is reliable, valid and easy to administer[54].

1.6.2.2 Interpreting MBI results

<u>Breakdown of the 22 items</u>

Burnout: questions 1.2.3.6.8.13.14.16.20.
Depersonalisation: questions 5.10.11.15.22.
Personal achievement: questions 4.7.9.12.17.18.19.21.
For each dimension, we add up the responses to the items that make it up and obtain scores.
Maslach and Jackson established limits for interpreting these scores as 'low', 'moderate' or 'high'.
Reference values set for the original MBI (MBI-HSS)

	MBI dimensions - HSS (MBI Original)		
Burnout score	EE	DP	AP
High	> 27	> 13	< 30
Moderate	17 - 26	7 - 12	31 - 36
Low	< 16	< 6	> 37

***Maslach Burnout Inventory Manual* [40].**

The French scale is the Fontaine MBI translation from the work by Canoui and Mauranges.

	MBI dimensions - French version		
Burnout score	EE	DP	AP
High	> 30	> 12	< 33
Moderate	18 - 29	6 - 11	34 - 39
Low	< 17	< 5	> 40

***MBI* (Fontaine translation) [15]**

- The level of emotional exhaustion is considered low, moderate or high for scores respectively set at < 17,18-29, > 30 ;
- For the degree of depersonalisation, the scores are respectively set at < 5, 6-11, > 12 ;
- For personal fulfilment, the scores are respectively set at < 33, 34-39, > 40 [3].

The personal fulfilment dimension is **inversely** related to the other two MBI dimensions: a low personal fulfilment score indicates a high level of burnout.

Depending on the number of dimensions affected, there are different stages of severity.

The degree of burnout is described as :

- Low: 1 dimension reached.
- Medium: 2/3 dimensions achieved.
- High: all 3 dimensions have been reached (high scores on the "emotional exhaustion" and "dehumanisation" subscales, combined with a low score on the "personal fulfilment" subscale).

For some authors[15] a moderate level of burnout can be measured by moderate scores on each scale, and the absence (or low level) of burnout can be measured by low scores on the emotional exhaustion and 'dehumanisation' scales, combined with a high score on personal fulfilment.

A high score on the EE subscale **or** the DP subscale **or** a low score on the AP subscale is sufficient to speak of burnout.

The simultaneous presence of the three dimensions of burnout in an individual is not necessary for a diagnosis [15].

According to Maslach, there is no global score; each of the 3 dimensions must be the subject of its own score, although some believe that it can be used globally in a single syndrome [55].

Maslach and Jackson consider burnout to be a continuous variable that expresses a degree of impairment, divided into low, medium and high.

They have not defined a clinical threshold that indicates the absence or presence of OO: a high score on the dimensions of emotional exhaustion and depersonalisation combined with a low score on personal fulfilment represents a high degree of OO [48].

I.7 DYNAMICS OF BURNOUT SYNDROME

Researchers are divided on the dynamics of OB. While some see it as a state, others take a more dynamic and evolutionary approach.

I.7.1 Burnout State

I.7.1.1 Definition

Let's start by recalling that *burnout* is, according to the most widely accepted definition (of which there are around fifty), a syndrome combining emotional and physical exhaustion, dehumanisation of the relationship with human beings and human activities, and a decline, or even disappearance, of the feeling of personal accomplishment, in response to a chronically stressful situation.

Most authors define burnout as an episode or state:

Freudenberger and Richelson in 1980, Maslach in 1982, Brill in 1984, Pines and Aronson in 1988.

The definition proposed by Brill in 1984 is less well known but very precise [22, 56] and has been translated by Zawieja as follows: "a dysphoric and dysfunctional state, linked to the professional expectations of an individual who does not present more marked psychopathological disorders, 1) who has previously demonstrated, under similar professional conditions, adequate performance and emotional reactions and 2) who, without external help or modification of his working conditions, is unable to return to his previous levels" [16].

I.7.1.2 Characteristics

Burnout can be recognised as a condition by five characteristics [22, 56]:

- Dysphoric elements predominate, including emotional exhaustion, fatigue and depression.
- Mental and behavioural symptoms are more important than physical signs.
- The third characteristic concerns the origin of the symptoms: burnout has its roots in the work environment.
- Symptoms occur in 'normal' people who have no previous mental pathology.
- The person displays negative behaviour towards others and becomes less effective, with low work performance.

The best known and most experimentally robust model of burnout as a 'state' is Maslach's *Attributional Environmental Model.*

This model has excellent theoretical and empirical foundations, and is considered by Maslach, Schaufeli and Leiter in 2001 to be the benchmark for research into the phenomenon. Burnout is defined as a multidimensional syndrome with three components: emotional exhaustion, depersonalisation and reduced personal fulfilment[25].

I.7.2 Burnout as a dynamic process

I.7.2.1 Descriptions of the phases of burnout

Several descriptions of the phases of burnout have been proposed:

1.7.2.1.1 Cherniss

- For Cherniss, the transaction between the individual and his environment develops in three stages[31] describing a stress-tension-coping-strategy-detachment process [15] :
- First of all, there is an imbalance between individual and organisational resources in the face of work demands [57].
- Work-related stress will therefore gradually develop, leading to a state of malaise that will be expressed by the employee's disengagement from his or her work.
- The strategies put in place to cope with these tensions, known as defensive coping, will be decisive in the development of burnout [25].

For Cherniss, burnout is "a process in which a previously committed professional disengages from his or her work in response to perceived stress and tension"[31].

1.7.2.1.2 Edelwich and Brodsky

- For Edelwich and Brodsky (1980), this is a process of 'disillusionment' with four distinct phases [57] :

1) Enthusiasm: This is the honeymoon phase. The employee will become over-invested in their work, idealising it and giving it an inordinate amount of importance. They are over-energetic and work long hours, even at home, to the detriment of their free time, neglecting

their private life and personal needs. This excess of enthusiasm leads them to devote themselves body and soul and to develop unrealistic expectations of their work [36, 38].

2) stagnation: the worker begins to realise that their professional investment is not rewarding and that work is not everything in this life.

Some discontent begins to surface, and the first symptoms of fatigue appear [36, 38].

3) frustration: professional difficulties become significant and skills are called into question. The subject becomes intolerant, less attentive to others and can no longer cope with the demands placed on them[25].

It is this feeling of frustration that is responsible for the physical, somatic, emotional and behavioural problems[36]. [58].

4) apathy: a state of depression and indifference in response to the many frustrations they face. This is a state of impasse and despair, with the subject thinking of suicide[58].

This stage is the very essence of burnout[25].

Edelwich and Brodsky define burnout as "a progressive decline in idealism, energy, ambition and participation, resulting from working conditions" [16].

I.7.2.1.3 Veniga and Spradley

- Veniga and Spradley in 1981 proposed an equivalent five-stage process:

1) Honeymoon corresponds to the first phase of the previous model.
2) A drop in energy and dissatisfaction characterise the second phase
3) The accentuation of avoidance strategies and symptoms of exhaustion correspond to the third phase.
4) At the fourth stage, the individual becomes pessimistic and tries to escape from work: this is the crisis.
5) The wall is the final stage, and burnout becomes inseparable from other disorders (addiction to drugs, alcohol, etc.)[25].

5.4.4.4.4 Lauderdale

- Lauderdale proposes three phases: "confusion", frustration and despair[18].

5.4.4.4.5 Freudenberger

- Freudenberger himself modified his initial 1974 concept [18], and in 1985 he and North presented burnout as an evolutionary process [15].

In his book, Canoui believes that his reflections and clinical experience have also led him to define burnout syndrome as a dynamic process[15].

5.4.4.4.6 Maslach and Schaufeli

In 1993, Maslach and Schaufeli suggested the following explanation for the link between state burnout and process burnout:

Burnout occurs when professional obligations become too great and too important, draining the individual's resources and energy.

To protect himself against the negative effects of this emotional exhaustion, he disinvests and disengages, which allows him to distance himself psychologically from users. The feeling of diminished personal fulfilment is reached when they become aware of the imbalance between their professional expectations and the reality on the ground[25].

I.8 FACTORS PREDISPOSING TO BURNOUT

Stress, psychosocial risks (RPS), burnout... so many semantic games in circulation, sometimes amplified by the megaphone of the media, as if they were the translation of a feeling towards their work that people don't always know how to express or of a malaise, as if these words alone said everything that hadn't been heard or understood until now. While these terms cover a wide range of situations experienced by workers, they all need to be analysed in terms of the work itself, the conditions under which it is carried out and the multiple relationships (customer relations, relations between colleagues, relations with the hierarchy, etc.) that are formed and dissolved in the workplace.

Today, burnout is seen as the result of complex, multifactorial, additional and interactive interactions between the individual and the environment, with a mutual and continuous influence between them[38].

However, according to some authors' studies, it is the organisational characteristics of the workplace that are responsible for the onset of burnout [26, 42].

I.8.1 Organisational and professional level

Maslach and his team have classified all the psychosocial factors at work responsible for burnout into six areas [42, 59]:

I.8.1.1 Psychosocial factors

1- The workload

This is the work stress most frequently associated with burnout. It can be quantitative (large amount of work under time pressure, number of hours worked) or qualitative (feeling unable to do the job properly).

Workload and time constraints are strongly linked to burnout.

As regards the qualitative aspect of work, studies have mainly focused on role conflict and role ambiguity, both of which show a relationship with burnout.

Role conflict occurs when the information required to do a job is contradictory, and role ambiguity occurs when this information is inadequate or insufficient to do the job well[25].Role conflict and role ambiguity are also called "role stressors"[60] and are strongly linked to the three dimensions of the MBI[61].

2- Control over work activity

Linked to a person's autonomy and decision-making power over their job; having little room for manoeuvre in the way they do their job, being unable to control it or situations increases the risk of burnout [26].

3- Community spirit

Refers to the social support that comes from hierarchy and colleagues, as well as the quality of human relations between individuals in the workplace.

4- Rewards

They may be extrinsic or intrinsic

The former refer to financial and social rewards (recognition and appreciation of efforts made), and the latter to the feeling of pride in doing a job and doing it well [26].the combined loss of these two categories of reward leads to burnout [42].the lack of reward is closely linked to the feeling of inefficiency [26].

5- Fairness and justice

Feelings of injustice can arise when there is inequity in the distribution of workload or pay, or when appraisals and promotions are inappropriate[62].

6- Value and ethics.

Losing a sense of purpose in one's work and feeling that one is doing a pointless job can be observed as a result of a lack of discussion with colleagues or management about the objectives to be achieved [43]. Feeling forced to do things that are unethical and at odds with your own values [26].

For the helping professions, in addition to organisational constraints, there are the emotional demands of the job [32].

❖ **Interaction between the six areas**

Researchers have looked into the relationship between these six areas.

Some studies suggest that the *value* dimension can act as a central mediator for the other dimensions.

However, there can be a significant individual difference: for example, some people may place more weight on rewards than on values, and may therefore be more affected by insufficient rewards than by value conflicts.

Another example is that an individual may be prepared to tolerate a heavy workload if, in return, they receive financial and social rewards, work in favourable conditions, maintain good relations with their colleagues and feel that their work is valued...

So we can't know exactly what individuals can tolerate.

Thus, the discrepancies that exist in these six domains at organisational level emphasise the importance to be attached to the individual, depending on how well he or she fits into these domains of working life [26].

For their part, Demerouti et al have proposed the **JD-R** (*Job Demands-Resources*) model, which groups occupational exposures relating to burnout into two categories: demands and resources.

I.8.1.2 Requirements-resources model

I.8.1.2.1 Requirements

Refers to different aspects of work (physical or organisational) that require sustained effort (physical or mental) and are therefore associated with a certain physiological and/or psychological cost (e.g. work overload, emotional demands, time pressure, poor working conditions [63, 64].

I.8.1.2.2 Resources

These include autonomy, social support and development opportunities.

Demands are linked to emotional exhaustion, while (lack of) resources are more closely linked to disengagement.

In the **JD-R** model, the development of burnout follows two processes:

The demands of the job lead to overwork, which in turn leads to exhaustion.

In the second process, a lack of resources leads to a feeling of failure and frustration, which in turn leads to withdrawal.

The long-term consequence of this withdrawal is disengagement from work[64].

I.8.2 At inter- and intra-individual level

Even if burnout has been identified in a professional context, and factors relating to work and its organisation will play an important role in the worker's suffering, two individuals with the same jobs and the same skills will not necessarily both suffer from burnout[25].

The ability to adapt to stressful work-related situations varies from one individual to another: for the same stressful situation, some will have psychological, emotional and functional reactions, while others will not[65].

Inter- and intra-individual variables are therefore important to study.

1.8.2.1 Inter-individual variables

These are mainly injustices experienced at work, situations of aggression, harassment, conflict, bullying, etc., which contribute to the onset of burnout[25].

1.8.2.2 Individual variables

There are individual differences that explain why a subject is more likely to encounter stressors, to be able to cope with stressful situations or to experience burnout.

1.8.2.2.1 Demographic factors

According to the literature, age, sex, level of education, marital status, number of children, length of work experience and lack of training show inconsistent relationships with burnout[66].

For some, burnout seems to affect (at least in the USA) young people under the age of 30 or 40, without much professional experience [22], since these people who tend to invest themselves excessively in their work feel that they are not getting back what they expected [65].

However, *these* results must be interpreted with caution, as it is possible that older subjects suffering from burnout left their jobs, and only those in good health remained.

Moreover, certain studies carried out in Europe, and more particularly in the Netherlands, have found that burnout is prevalent in the elderly[22].

1.8.2.2.2 Personality

There are personality traits that more or less predict and explain an individual's behaviour.

Mc Crae and Costa in 1990 proposed the following definition: "personality traits are dimensions describing individual differences in tendencies to manifest coherent and systematic patterns of thoughts, emotions and actions"[67]. Some authors believe that personality is one of the most important factors in the onset of burnout[68].

I.8.2.2.2.1 The Big Five

Numerous studies have been carried out in recent years to classify personalities.

Five factors have been identified as the FFM (Five Factor Model) or "Big Five" [69].

This five-factor model has unquestionably become the reference model and has been the subject of a great deal of research in recent years [67].

The "Big Five" were initially numbered as follows: (I) Intervention (or Extraversion), (II) Agreeable, (III) Conscientious (or Reliable), (IV) Emotional Stability (vs. Neuroticism), and (V) Culture. Factor V was later renamed "Intellect" and then Open[70].

These personality traits are considered to be stable over time at the individual level [71].

a- Extraversion

To be likely to experience positive emotions, such as cheerfulness, enthusiasm and optimism, to have self-confidence with a more favourable and positive view of the level of personal effectiveness, and to appreciate the interpersonal links created in the workplace [72].

b- Pleasantness

To be cooperative, attentive, trusting and sympathetic towards others[73].these agreeable workers behave in such a way as to elicit favourable reactions in their social environment[74]. Their adaptability enables them to have a positive view of work, and their good humour and tendency to be affectionate and warm lead to successful interpersonal relationships [72].

c- The conscientious postman

These individuals are less likely to experience emotional exhaustion because of their work ethic and perseverance, according to Costa and Mc Crae. Given their nature of wanting to carry out work efficiently and with good performance, it is not surprising to see a high degree of personal fulfilment on their part[72].

d- Neuroticism

This trait reflects emotional instability.

It is defined by negative feelings such as anxiety, sadness, frustration, guilt and nervous tension[74].neuroticism is strongly linked to the onset of burnout[75, 76], particularly emotional exhaustion[77].

e- Openness to experience

Be curious, creative, imaginative and ready for new experiences and ideas [74].

Work situations that contain uncertainty or ambiguity should not arouse feelings of unease and apprehension in these individuals; on the contrary, they look forward to such opportunities.

As a result, they are less likely to be emotionally drained if they experience frustration or anxiety [72].

I.8.2.2.2.2 Hardiness

The term *hardiness*, described by Suzanne Kobasa and translated as endurance, solidity, psychic robustness or even boldness, refers to a personality characteristic designed to protect the individual from stressful life events.

Of all the personal resources, hardiness seems to be recognised as the most powerful resource for coping with stress[15].

Individuals with this trait tend to believe that they can control the events that happen to them; they generally perceive stressors as challenges rather than threats[74].

According to Maddi and Kobasa, there are three dimensions of hardiness

- Commitment
- Mastery
- The challenge

a- The sense of commitment is the individual's tendency to become totally involved in the various situations they encounter, to feel concerned by what is happening to them or to those around them, and to commit easily to action, thus giving meaning to their experience.

For him, work is a pleasure, and events, objects and people in his environment are considered interesting.

Being committed requires a belief in being pro-active, a tendency to take action and move forward.

b- A sense of control: as opposed to powerlessness, this is a belief that the individual can positively influence events and change situations through action and reflection.

They have confidence in their decision-making ability and believe that the actions they take at work will enable them to achieve their objectives.

c- The meaning of the challenge

The individual perceives change as a challenge, as an important stimulus for growth and development.

Having a sense of challenge means being easily open to change, enjoying variety and evolution in work, and being focused on self-fulfilment rather than stability and security[15].

I.8.2.2.2.3 Type A personality

The work of two cardiologists, Friedman and Rosenman (1974), described this type of personality.

According to them, type A individuals are more vulnerable to occupational stress and have a higher incidence of developing heart problems.

These individuals are very involved in their work, are impatient and have a pronounced taste for competition [57]. They tend to be aggressive and hostile, easily angered, and may perceive even minor affronts as major injustices, which deprives them of the support of those around them [74].

The meta-analysis by Alarcon and colleagues found an association between type A personality and the dimension "loss of personal fulfilment"[74].

I.8.2.2.2.4 Self-esteem

According to Brockner (1988), self-esteem at work refers to an individual's self-assessment of competence and personal value in the workplace. It indicates the degree to which they perceive themselves to be capable and effective.

People with low self-esteem tend to depersonalise their clients and work colleagues, and experience feelings of ineffectiveness in their relationships with others.

These individuals may also have few psychological resources to help them cope with the stress factors that lead to burnout[78].

According to Tharenou (1979), people with low self-esteem show more anxiety, depression and neurotic behaviour, perform their work less effectively under stress, have reduced social skills, lack initiative and tend to have low aspirations[78].

I.8.2.2.3 Beliefs

a- Locus of control: LOC

The locus theory, or "places of reinforcement control", developed in 1966 by Rotter is based on the fact that the individual attributes responsibility for his successes or failures to internal factors (under the influence of his will to control his destiny) or to external factors (chance, fate, other people and not as the result of his own actions)[15].

He believes that it is his own behaviour that determines the consequences of events, known as reinforcements[79].

Studies using the Locus of Control or Rotter scale show that the internal LOC has a protective effect against stress, making it a success factor, whereas people with an 'external control' type have a pattern of anxious, helpless and depressive behaviour, and are therefore more emotionally vulnerable.

However, the 'internal-control' individual is not all good: he is more resistant to external influences, but less able to withstand the changes demanded of him, particularly in the organisation of work [15, 30].

b- Self-efficacy

Bandura introduced the theory of self-efficacy, which refers to an individual's belief in his or her ability to organise and carry out the behaviours required to manage future situations.

This belief of being effective influences the way these individuals think, feel, motivate and act[80].

c- Religion :

It can be a resource for the individual and a means of adapting to difficult situations (coping). However, it can also be a source of stress when faced with a situation where you are powerless to help others, creating feelings of guilt and shame[37].

I.8.2.2.4 Individual coping strategies

According to Lazarus and Folkman, *coping* refers to the set of constantly changing cognitive and behavioural efforts aimed at controlling specific demands (internal or external) that are assessed as threatening or exceeding the individual's resources[25].

There are two coping strategies:

- the passive strategy :

The subject avoids problems, withdraws into himself, isolates himself, withdraws and resigns himself to his fate. This strategy is relatively effective and does not sufficiently mobilise the individual's fighting spirit.

- active strategy :

The subject confronts problems with the ability to re-evaluate them in a positive way, and the conviction of being able to act decisively on them. They express their emotions verbally and do not hesitate to enter into relationships with others[15].

I.8.2.2.5 Career options

Everyone has expectations of their work: financial reward, social recognition, acquisition of skills, etc.

So work is a way of achieving goals, boosting self-efficacy, self-esteem and material comfort.

To better understand these expectations and their impact on the individual, Cherniss developed the notion of *career* orientation [47].

There are four main areas of focus:

a- The social activist: cares little about their status or the security of their job and seeks to bring about social change through what they do. An idealist, work represents more of a commitment than a job.

b- The careerist: seeks success, prestige, responsibility, financial security, social recognition... Concerned with social respectability and promotion, they strive to obtain external reinforcement.

c- The craftsman: values the development of his skills, wants to acquire new knowledge, maintains a certain independence and tries to test new methods.

Work is an opportunity for them to practise their skills or develop them through new experiences.

d- The egoist: the most important thing for him is to satisfy his private life, and he makes little commitment to his work. Leisure and family take precedence over work, which is merely a means of making a profit in their extra-professional life.

In his study of French self-employed doctors, Truchot found that it was the careerists and egoists who were most at risk of burnout, while the activists and craftsmen were the most protected [47].

I.8.2.3 Other individual factors

In 2003, Fauteux identified seven main individual factors which, according to him, are likely to lead to burnout:

1- perfectionism
2- low self-esteem
3- idealism
4- performance pressure
5- predisposition to anxiety
6- assertiveness difficulties
7- difficulties linked to stress management[81].

Freudenberger and Richelson also described the people who could develop this syndrome:

These are men and women who see themselves as dynamic, charismatic, competent and who have an idealised image of themselves. These individuals are dedicated and committed to everything they do. The reality check eventually leads to the development of burnout[27].

<u>In conclusion</u>

The individual vulnerability factors that may contribute to or encourage the onset of burnout are [26] :

- Low level of hardiness
- External LOC
- Passive adaptation style

- Lower self-esteem
- Big Five neuroticism
- Type A behaviour.

I.9 LIMITS OF THE SYNDROME

To date, burnout syndrome has lacked homogeneity. Psychiatrists refer to it as a non-specific symptomatology that may cover several diagnostic fields: adjustment disorders, anxiety disorders, depressive disorders and somatisation [15].

Given the importance of this psychosocial phenomenon, we will try to :

- to situate burnout within the framework of occupational psychopathology
- detail stress and investigate its relationship to burnout
- identify the relationships and differences between burnout and certain psychiatric conditions.

1.9.1 Burnout and occupational psychopathology

From "work fatigue" to "burnout

The term "occupational psychopathology" was first proposed in 1952 by P. Sivadon, and generally refers to a body of theoretical knowledge concerning the pathogenic repercussions of work on an individual's mental health[17].

It can be defined as "the dynamic analysis of the psychological processes mobilised by the subject's confrontation with the reality of work". "Dynamic" means that the centre of gravity of the investigation is the **conflicts** which may arise as a result of the encounter between a subject with a particular history pre-existing this encounter, and a work situation whose characteristics are fixed independently of the subject's will[82].

Most researchers agree that the theories of Christophe Dejours (a psychiatrist, psychoanalyst and occupational physician) have undeniably given new impetus to this discipline.

For Dejours, the study of suffering due to psychic load is the privileged place of investigation for work psychopathology[15]. In 1980, he published a work entitled "travail : usure mentale. Essai de psychopathologie du travail", in which he described the unseen suffering and internalisation of work constraints, particularly in the working world[18].

There are different approaches to occupational psychopathology:

1.9.1.1 The sociological approach

It is essentially social conflicts at work (class struggle, power relations within the company and within society as a whole) that are at the root of the pathology.

The conditions and organisation of work bear witness to social pathology[15].

1.9.1.2 The psychiatric approach

In this approach, work can reveal the pathology.

However, while work can be a source of adjustment problems, it can also become a therapeutic tool, helping to rehabilitate patients by enhancing their self-esteem.

So work has a dual impact: it can be a source of suffering, or a source of balance[15].

1.9.1.3 The psychoanalytical approach

Psychoanalysis takes account of the endogenous sources of suffering in the individual.

According to Dejours, the origins of the latter lie in the psychic organisation that develops during the first three to five years of life.

Work is therefore not seen as the cause of psychological suffering, but as the revelation of an underlying fault that has existed since the first years of life. This is why Dejours says of this approach that "psychoanalytic radicalism disqualifies the psychopathology of work"[18].

The burnout hypothesis is not totally at odds with this approach, and may be a possible interpretation. But the other hypothesis is that burnout can be observed in a normal individual, and it is in this individual's ability to *cope* that the psychopathology of the onset of maladaptation will be discussed[15].

1.9.1.4 The Pavlovian approach

The Pavlovian approach is the study of the behavioural stereotypes of a person.

The "contamination" of non-work life by work automatisms [15].

J. Bégoin and L. Le Guillant focused on the pathogenic consequences of work on individuals. Their study took place at the French Post Office during the 1950s and focused on the work of telephone operators, leading them to identify a specific syndrome linked to the material and psychological conditions of work: the "neurosis of telephone operators and mechanographers".

The authors' analysis of the disorders presented by telephone operators, and in particular the "common subjective syndrome of nervous fatigue", refers to Pavlov's model of experimental neurosis[17].

Another example is the film "Modern Times", in which the famous actor Charlie Chaplin attempts to unscrew two huge black buttons from a lady's suit, continuing the stereotypical gestures he was making on the bolt assembly line he had been working on a few minutes earlier.

However, the repetition of these low-skilled tasks does not allow a sufficiently diversified psychopathological approach to work to explain these disorders[15].

1.9.1.5 The stress theory approach

Stress plays a central role in occupational psychopathology and is a key factor in the onset of burnout [30] (it will therefore be discussed in more detail below).

All these descriptions foreshadow subsequent developments around the notion of stress and the return of 'fatigue' under the name of burnout[17].

Burnout, by bringing a particular dimension to the repercussions of work on human beings, serves work psychopathology, and approaches to psychopathology are used to analyse the factors involved in the onset of burnout[15].

1.9.2 Burnout and Stress

There is a particular interaction between stress at work and the development of burnout syndrome. To understand the relationship between stress and burnout, it is first necessary to situate the concepts of stress.

We will define burnout and set out the various explanatory models on which most research into burnout has been based.

I.9.2.1 Stress

In eighteenth-century England, "stress" meant distress linked to oppression, hardship, deprivation, adversity... [15].

The word "stress" derives from the Latin stringere [83]: to embrace, squeeze, hurt. It gave rise in Old French to the term *estrece*: oppression, narrowness [79] and in Middle English to its doublet *distress* (détresse): misfortune, difficulty, affliction. [15].

In the field of physics, it refers to the stress exerted on a material which initially resists, but as the stress persists, the material deforms and breaks[83, 84].Hans Selye, a Canadian doctor of Hungarian origin, put the concept on a scientific footing and spread it almost worldwide[15].His work from the 1930s onwards was of major importance in the development and popularity of this concept[85].

According to his approach, stress cannot be avoided; it is a normal, non-specific response by the body to a stimulus.

It describes eustress (good stress) when the effects of stressors are positive, and distress (negative stress) if the effects are harmful.

Individuals do not all react in the same way to stress; this is not surprising, since no two individuals in the world are identical[86], each being conditioned by genetic factors, psychological characteristics and the social environment[57].It is not so much what happens to the person, but the way in which they react that counts in its genesis[86].

Selye drew attention to the work of Claude Bernard, which showed the importance of maintaining a constant internal environment, and the principle of the body's return to homeostasis after exposure to a stressor described by Cannon[87].

In addition to Cannon's studies on homeostasis, the notion of 'fight or flight', which he considered an essential reaction for survival, was also developed. In his view, stress is a break in the normal physiological state, with a disruption in homeostasis.

Moreover, this researcher is considered a great source of inspiration for contemporary authors researching this subject[83].

1.9.2.1.1 Stimulus-response model

When a living organism is exposed to continuous stress over long periods of time, it necessarily goes through three phases, referred to by Selye as the "**General Adaptation Syndrome" (GAS)**: alarm reaction, resistance stage and exhaustion stage (research was carried out on rats) [87] :

a- alarm reaction: adrenaline discharge with a series of neurovegetative reactions

- increase in blood pressure,
- increased heart rate,
- perspiration,
- various muscular reactions,
- depletion of energy reserves (glucose and lipids) [88].

If the stress factor (stressor) is so severe that continued exposure is incompatible with life, the organism will die within a few hours or days during this phase[86].

b- Resistance or adaptation stage: no organism can be kept in a constant state of alert. This phase is characterised by the disappearance or reduction of the initial symptoms; the body has reached optimal adaptation.

c- exhaustion stage : After even more prolonged exposure to stress factors, the acquired adaptation is lost and physiological resources become insufficient; the terminal stage then occurs[86]. In rats, failure to adapt results in death from haemorrhagic digestive ulceration and in humans, various physical and/or psychological pathologies may occur[88].

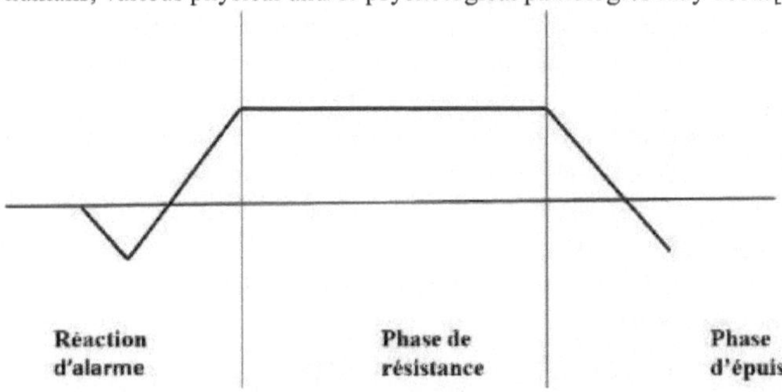

The General Adaptation Syndrome (after Selye, 1979)

The General Adaptation Syndrome

Work carried out in the wake of the Cannon and Selye studies has shown that exposure to environmental conditions produces hormonal changes that can lead to physiological and psychological problems.

Biomedical research has enabled us to understand how the brain controls the functioning of hormones and the neurovegetative system.

Several neuroregulators involved in adaptation reactions have been identified (catecholamines and endorphins).

According to some researchers, more than a dozen neuroactive substances are involved in the neurophysiological process of reacting to stress[57].

This initial conception of stress corresponded to linear **stimuli/response models**; physiological responses of the organism to an aggressive agent (Cannon, Selye) which tends to disrupt the individual's homeostasis.

To restore this balance, it responds via the neurohormonal systems (sympathetic, medullary-adrenal and hypothalamic-pituitary-adrenal)[15].

The main limitation of these models is that they take into account neither inter-individual variations nor the psychological component, and therefore define the individual as passive in the face of this aggressive agent [79].

This linear stimulus/response model has been abandoned in favour of a transactional model[15].

1.9.2.1.2 Transactional models

1.9.2.1.2.1 Karasek Job Demands-Control model

In this Job Demands-Control (JD-C) model[89], the degree of tension felt by the worker results from the interaction between "psychological demand" (psychological demands of the job) and "decision-making autonomy (or latitude)" at work.

Professional demands are defined by Karasek and Theorell (1990) as the psychological costs necessary to carry out one's work[90].

a- Psychological demand: refers to the performance of tasks, the quantity and complexity of the work, unforeseen tasks, time constraints, frequent interruptions, etc. This is the psychological workload.

b- Decision latitude: the ability to choose how to work, to participate in decision-making, to use one's skills and to be creative.

By combining the two characteristics of psychological demand and decision-making ability, we can identify the following four types of situation: (see table or diagram)

- The work is relaxed, if there are low psychological demands and a high degree of decision-making autonomy.
- The work is active or dynamic, if there is a high level of psychological demand combined with a high degree of decision-making autonomy.
- On the other hand, a job is passive if there is an association between low psychological demand and low decision-making autonomy.
- The situation most prone to ***job strain*** is the combination of low decision-making latitude and high psychological demand.

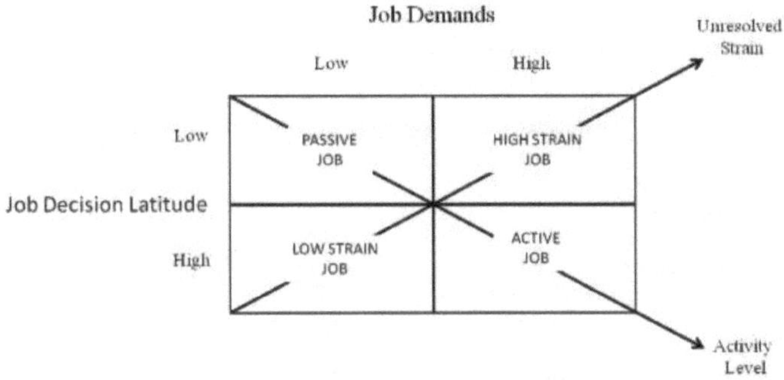

Job strain model (de Karasek) 1979

		Psychological demands	
		Low	High
Decision-making latitude	Low	Passive work	Tense or overloaded work: job strain
	High	Relaxed work	Active work

Karasek requirement-control model

Work constraint can be improved by increasing decision latitude, independently of changes in psychological demand. It should be noted that it is not the level of stress that is measured, but rather exposure to stress risk factors (such as a tense situation in the work environment)[89].
In 1985, Karasek developed and published a valid and recognised tool for assessing the constraints of the psychosocial environment at work. It is called the Job Content Questionnaire (JCQ) or Karasek Questionnaire [91].
Initially, the model proposed was two-dimensional, but in 1990 Karasek and Theorell introduced a third dimension: social support at work from superiors and colleagues.
A work situation is potentially stressful if it combines: high work demands, little or no control over one's own work and little social support from colleagues or superiors[92].

1.9.2.1.2.2 Siegrist's effort-reward model (1990)

This theoretical concept has been proposed to assess the harmful effects of work-related stress on health: the effort-reward imbalance model.
This model is based on the reciprocity of exchanges in professional life: efforts made, rewards expected.
In fact, an imbalance between major efforts at work and little reward in return leads to a particularly stressful situation.

- There are two types of effort:
- extrinsic effort: linked to the pressure and demands of the job.
- Intrinsic effort: high need for control, employee motivation linked to excessive commitment, etc.
- The awards are :

- the money

- esteem
- status control (it is weak in the case of lack of promotion prospects, job insecurity, etc.)[93].

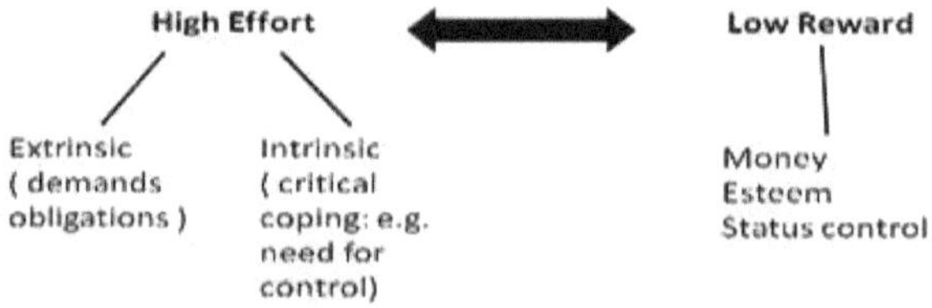

The effort -reword imbalance model at work

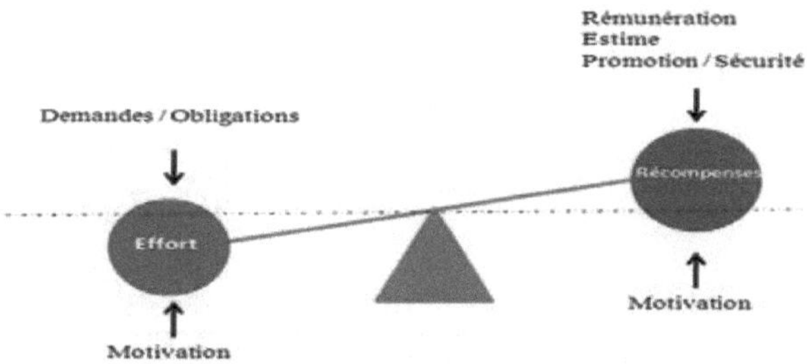

Balance effort-récompense du modèle de Siegrist

1.9.2.1.2.3 Transactional model by Lazarus and Folkman (1984)

This concept is based on **cognitive assessment**.

In this model, the person and the environment are considered to be in a dynamic, mutually reciprocal and bidirectional relationship.

Stress can arise when this relationship is assessed by the person as exceeding their resources, and endangering their well-being.

The theory identifies two mediators that intervene and modulate the stress reaction: cognitive appraisal and coping strategies.

a- Cognitive evaluation is a process whereby the individual assesses whether a particular encounter with the environment is relevant to his or her well-being and, if so, in what way.

There are two types of cognitive evaluation: primary and secondary.

- primary assessment: the person analyses the situation (personality characteristics, values, goals and beliefs may come into play).
- secondary assessment: the person assesses what needs to be done to manage or prevent the situation.

Various coping options are evaluated, such as changing the situation, accepting it, seeking more information or refraining from acting impulsively.

b- Coping refers to the individual's cognitive and behavioural efforts to manage (reduce, minimise, control or tolerate) the internal and external demands of the person-environment transaction which is assessed as exceeding the individual's resources.

There are 2 types of Coping:

- Active coping: strategy centred on the problem, with an attempt to deal with it and efforts to change the situation.

- Passive coping: strategy centred on emotions and distancing, self-control, seeking social support, avoidance and attempts to regulate emotional reactions.

Cognitive appraisal and *coping* are therefore transactional variables, which means that they do not refer to the environment or the person, but to the integration of the two in a given transaction [94].

1.9.2.1.2.4 Hobfoll's resource conservation model

Hobfoll's resource conservation theory, developed in 1989, is a model that may better reflect current knowledge of stress. This model aims to fill the gaps that exist in biological and cognitive theories.

This theory proposes a motivational model, and is now one of the most studied theories of stress[95].the basic principle is that individuals seek to create a world that gives them pleasure and success[84].to do this, they strive to obtain, conserve, protect and develop resources, and stress occurs when these resources are threatened with loss or are lost, or when individuals fail to obtain them[96].

Different types of resources in Western countries are grouped into four main groups:

- objects: house, car, jewellery, spare cash, etc.
- conditions: good health, a successful relationship, stable employment, etc.
- personal characteristics: optimism, sense of humour, ability to plan, etc.
- elements that encourage dynamism: knowledge, communication skills, being appreciated, having friends, etc.

These resources are interconnected; the gain or loss of one of them will have repercussions on the others in the different groups (e.g. the death of a spouse will have repercussions on optimism, the education of children and family stability, the acquisition of objects, etc.).

The loss of resources is felt much more by the individual than a gain, and in a disproportionate way, which is the first principle of the theory. This leads us to the second principle of the theory, which states that the individual will constantly try to enrich his resources by investing others, thus adopting a long-term perspective to conserve his resources and possibly compensate for the possibility of future losses in the interests of well-being[95].

In burnout, the individual has few resources which he uses continuously, avoiding investing more and thus running the risk of losing his last reserves and becoming exhausted. Hobfoll's theory of resource conservation therefore provides a perspective that reflects our current understanding of stress.

It is a testable model, which exhaustively explains the individual's behaviour in stressful circumstances. This model is very interesting and is increasingly used in burnout research [84].

1.1.1 .2 Burnout-Stress relationship

Definitions of burnout often refer to stress. These two concepts are difficult to separate and the same causes are often found in both cases.

For Farber, burnout can be seen "as the final stage in a progression of futile attempts to cope with a variety of **stressful conditions** perceived as negative".

For Cherniss and Edelwich, burnout is a psychological withdrawal from work in response to excessive **stress**[57].

Stress is a term that refers to the process of temporary adaptation accompanied by physical and psychological symptoms.

Burnout, on the other hand, can be seen as the final stage of a breakdown in adaptation resulting from a prolonged imbalance between demands and resources[97].

Burnout is prolonged occupational stress resulting from demands in the workplace that exceed an individual's resources.

In Selye's work, exposure to a stressor leads to the general adaptation syndrome with its three phases: alarm, resistance and exhaustion.

In this final phase, and after prolonged exposure to stress, physiological resources are exhausted and irreversible damage is done to the body. Referring to the adaptation syndrome, Etzion defines burnout as a latent process of psychological erosion resulting from prolonged exposure to occupational stress[56].

Burnout is therefore an illness characteristic of the helping relationship, which encompasses and goes beyond stress[98].

According to Canoui, burnout is therefore second to prolonged, repeated and long-term stress, which is part of a process of maladaptive reactions on the part of the individual:

Burnout is the result of chronic stress. It is a long and evolving phenomenon: it would be totally inappropriate to use this term after an acute event [15].

1.9.3 Burnout and job dissatisfaction

There is a distinction to be made between job dissatisfaction and burnout. While burnout implies dissatisfaction at work, the reverse is not true.

In their book, Canoui and Mauranges quote *Bédard and Duquette*, who state that "job dissatisfaction occurs when there is a mismatch between an individual's needs and the intrinsic and extrinsic factors associated with the job (...) Like burnout, dissatisfaction is a negative psychological experience experienced by the individual and linked to the work environment. The loss of a sense of accomplishment at work is a characteristic observed in people who are dissatisfied with their work (...) But emotional exhaustion, physical fatigue and the dehumanisation of relationships are not manifestations of job dissatisfaction (...) Finally, dissatisfaction can be expressed in relation to any type of work, whereas burnout syndrome is linked to work that aims to help people"[15].

So burnout is not just about dissatisfaction at work[18].

Indeed, if we take Malsach's three dimensions, namely emotional exhaustion, dehumanisation and loss of personal fulfilment, we do indeed find a decline or loss of self-fulfilment for people dissatisfied at work, but the first two dimensions are absent.

On the other hand, dissatisfaction at work can be seen in all professions, whereas burnout is limited, according to several authors, to professions whose purpose is to help.

1.9.4 Burnout and psychiatric disorders.

1.9.4.1 Burnout and depression

Empirical research suggests that burnout and depression are distinct entities [99], but they share a number of common features [3, 100-102], particularly in severe forms of burnout [55, 99] and in vulnerable individuals (type A personality, neuroticism, LOC, etc.) [99, 103].

- The similarities between depression and burnout :
- In the emotional exhaustion dimension of burnout, the subject presents sadness and fatigue, in depersonalisation, there is a characteristic of social withdrawal, and in the third dimension "decline in personal accomplishment", there is a decline in feelings of self-efficacy and powerlessness. All these symptoms are present in depression[100].
- Depressive feelings and various somatic complaints may suggest a diagnosis of masked depression or essential depression[15].
- In 1984, Meier showed a strong correlation between the burnout assessment scale and the depression scale [15, 18].

For these reasons, some psychiatrists have reduced burnout to a clinical form of depression [15].

- Burnout can be a precursor to full-blown major depression, but there is a distinction to be made between "depression" and "burnout" [15] :
- While in the case of depression, depressive symptoms affect all areas of life, during burnout they are most often limited to the professional sphere[103].
- Psychological and/or motor slowing is absent
- Although burnout can lead to a depressive illness, it occurs in people with no history of psychopathological disorders.
- The factors triggering burnout are usually multidimensional and cannot be clearly identified, which means we cannot equate it with reactive depression[15].

In general, if the criteria for diagnosing depression are rigorously adhered to, they are not all met in the case of burnout.

1.9.4.2 Burnout and anxiety

Anxiety disorders are defined by precise psychiatric criteria. Their semiology, assessment and treatment methods are well defined. Burnout is not an illness, but a reaction to chronic stress. However, like depression, burnout can also lead to a genuine anxiety disorder[15].

These overlaps between burnout and anxiety may probably be due to the fact that a high level of emotional exhaustion increases anxiety levels in stressful situations, making individuals more fragile [25].

1.9.4.3 Burnout and somatisation

The "concept" of somatisation suffers from a lack of precision and confusion as to its meaning [104, 105].

The term was coined in the 1920s by the psychoanalyst Wilhelm Stekel, who is credited in psychiatric literature as the originator of the concept.

In 1968, Lipowski proposed a revision of the term, giving it the following definition:

"the tendency to have, conceptualise and/or communicate psychological states or contents in the form of bodily sensations, functional changes or somatic metaphors" [104].

According to the DSM-IV, this is a multi-symptomatic disorder that begins before the third decade of life and persists for several years, often fluctuating. It combines painful body sites with gastrointestinal, sexual and pseudoneurological symptoms:

history of pain affecting at least four body sites (headache, abdominal pain, spinal pain, etc.) or bodily functions (urination, sexual intercourse, menstruation, etc.) with two gastrointestinal symptoms (nausea, abdominal bloating, vomiting, etc.), at least one sexual or genital symptom (metrorrhagia, erectile dysfunction, etc.) and at least one neurological symptom (paresis, laryngeal spasm, psychogenic non-epileptic seizures, etc.).

The patient's complaints are not objectified either by the clinical examination, which is normal, or by complementary investigations[105]. These disorders are beyond the control of the subject's will, and the reasons for them are unconscious [15].

Conversion refers to one or more productive or deficient symptoms affecting voluntary motor, sensory and sensory functions, in the absence of any objectivised organic suffering on clinical examination and complementary tests[105].

The hypochondriac is obsessed by his state of health, and is convinced that he is suffering from a serious illness which the doctors are unable to diagnose, despite the reassuring results of the additional tests carried out [105].

In the case of burnout, somatisations occupy a special place, as they are a very frequent

source of complaint among burned-out subjects.
However, it should be noted that none of the clinical signs is specific to burnout, and that unlike the hypochondriac, the individual is not afraid of suffering from any illness [15].
1.9.4.4 Burnout: an adaptation disorder
Burnout does not appear in the nosography of mental illnesses. There is resistance in the psychiatric world to the adoption of this nosographic term [57]. It is not officially diagnosed in the reference medical classifications, namely the 10th edition of the International Statistical Classification of Diseases and Related Health Problems (ICD-10) of the World Health Organisation (WHO), and the Diagnostic *and* Statistical *Manual of Mental Disorders* (DSM) of the American Psychiatric Association (APA). Even the DSM-V published in May 2013[106] did not include it.
It should be noted that in the ICD 10, "overwork" is mentioned as a state of exhaustion under **Z73.0** [107].
It is clear from these classifications that this syndrome is not characterised by a single, precise "clinical diagnosis", which mentions both well-defined symptoms and causes[43].
Some authors believe that it is legitimate to consider the burnout syndrome as a clinical form of an **adjustment disorder** [15, 25] or as a model of misconduct that is increasingly accepted socially [57].
It cannot be a diagnostic category, but rather a diagnosis of elimination and retrospection [15].

1.10MEDICINE AND DOCTORS

1.10.1 Medicine

In Algeria, there is executive decree no. 94-219 of 14 Safar 1415 corresponding to 23 July 1994 amending and supplementing decree no. 71-215 of 25 August 1971 on the organisation of medical studies[108] (appendix 1).
It stipulates that :

- The duration of studies for the degree of Doctor of Medicine is seven (7) years.
- Candidates for the diploma of Doctor of Medicine must hold a scientific baccalaureate diploma, the series of which is set by the Minister for Higher Education, or a foreign qualification recognised as equivalent.
- The studies leading to the degree of Doctor of Medicine are divided into two cycles and an internship:
- The first or pre-clinical cycle comprises the 1st, 2nd and 3rd years,
- the second or clinical cycle comprises the 4th, 5th and 6th years
- a one-year full-time internship in various university hospital departments and, where appropriate, in public health structures, the list of which is determined by the ministers responsible for higher education and health.

The practical and supervised courses that make up the two cycles and the internship are compulsory.

1.10.2 The doctor

1.10.2.1 Specific characteristics of medical students
Students who opt to study medicine are usually good students who have obtained their baccalauréat with a good mark.
They were generally excellent at school and went into medicine for a variety of reasons.
These include the influence of a supportive family environment, the physician's aspiration to social status and prestige, interest in this science and in human beings, and personal or family experience of illness.

However, many of the students who go into medicine have no real knowledge or awareness of the investment of time and energy required by these studies, or of the stamina and mental strength that are indispensable for coping with the long, selective and competitive study of medicine.

And the gap between the medical student's ideal and the day-to-day reality of the profession can be a painful disillusionment.

Given the lack of personal satisfaction, the young doctor will nourish the hope of being rewarded for his work at a later date, through future professional fulfilment and a better life balance[30].

1.10.2.2 The doctor-patient relationship

The contract between doctor and patient is the provision of care. However, the duty to provide proof of information and to transmit medical records calls into question the doctor's commitment, which is tacitly based on mutual trust. These new legal obligations disrupt the usual modes of communication and make the relationship more difficult.

On the other hand, medical studies have not prepared doctors to come face to face with suffering, illness and death. Nor do they teach the need for administrative and managerial skills. A doctor's vocation is to provide care, not to manage paperwork. On a daily basis, doctors experience relational tensions and emotions that need to be managed[109].

1.10.2.3 The sick doctor

When doctors fall ill, their professional status prevents them from seeing themselves as such: they are patients like no others. They are the first to deny that they are suffering, to ignore their discomfort, to hide their problems from their colleagues and to put off seeking medical help, often worsening their prognosis.

In the majority of cases, the doctor will not benefit from a typical care pathway and will resort to self-diagnosis and self-medication. They often feel embarrassed to consult a colleague for fear of upsetting them and exposing their weaknesses.

What's more, sick doctors find it difficult to accept the role of patient and are tempted to resume their status as doctors.

In addition, when they do consult a doctor, the follow-up is rarely regular. The financial aspect can also represent an obstacle to follow-up, since it is common for doctors not to charge their colleagues. The complex status of the sick doctor can give rise to a serious public health problem[79].

1.10.2.4 Burnout among GPs

As GPs are the first to be consulted for many health problems, both preventive and curative, the impact of their suffering on society will be felt both in terms of the quality of the care they provide and the continuity of their care for patients. In severe cases, the doctor may have to suspend his or her practice temporarily or even permanently[8].

1.10.2.5 Medical error and suicide

The suffering of a carer faced with a medical error or legal challenge can be so great that it can lead to suicide.

In the usual cultural context, an adverse event related to healthcare is perceived as being generated by a bad doctor rather than by infallible medicine[110].

In France in 2003, the Medical Council sounded the alarm about the abnormally high number of suicides by doctors in the Vaucluse department (11 suicides out of the 22 deaths recorded among practising doctors).

Other statistics also confirm this major cause of death among doctors in developed countries

[15].

1.11PREVENTING BURNOUT

According to Maslach, interventions need to be designed around the three dimensions of burnout. In other words, how can a particular strategy reduce the likelihood of **emotional exhaustion**, prevent the tendency **to depersonalise** and/or improve the sense of **personal accomplishment**?

This proposed strategy effectively addresses the phenomenon of burnout, and establishes relevant criteria for determining the effectiveness of the intervention[111].

As early as 1948, the World Health Organisation (WHO) defined three types of prevention, corresponding to successive states of the disease, and ranging from the means to be implemented to prevent the onset of pathologies to their treatment, possibly by preparing the social reintegration of patients [112].

- Primary prevention :

This is the set of actions designed to reduce the incidence of a disease in a population, in other words, to reduce the risk of new cases appearing.

- Secondary prevention

Its aim is to reduce the prevalence of a disease in a population. At this stage, therefore, the aim is to take action at the very beginning of the onset of the disorder or pathology, in order to halt its development or eliminate the risk factors.

Screening, diagnosis and treatment to prevent disease progression are essential components of secondary prevention.

- Tertiary prevention

At this stage, it is important to reduce the prevalence of chronic disability or recurrence in a population, and therefore to reduce the complications, disability and relapses caused by the disease.

Prevention aims to rehabilitate the patient in three ways: medically, socially and psychologically.

Quick (1992) applied this prevention approach to mental health risks in the workplace:

- Eliminating or reducing stress factors at work is considered **primary** prevention, as the intention is to reduce the incidence of new cases of stress.
- Interventions designed to help people manage or cope with these stressors at work are referred to as **secondary** prevention measures, as they aim to reduce the prevalence of stress.
- Intervention to treat individuals who are already suffering as a result of
exposure to these stress factors in the workplace is referred to as **tertiary** prevention[111].

The same tools are used to prevent burnout as are used to prevent stress and psychosocial risks. All three types of prevention (primary, secondary and tertiary) are therefore necessary[35].

The primary approach involves acting on the work environment, while the secondary or tertiary approach focuses on the individual.

In the literature, prevention measures focused on the individual encompass both treatment and prevention of its occurrence, and the distinction between the two approaches (secondary and tertiary) is not very clear.

In many cases, the same strategy has been proposed both to improve burnout and to prevent it[111].

In the section dealing with "factors predisposing to burnout", we found that these factors can be observed at organisational, inter-individual and individual levels, so action needs to be

taken at all three levels to prevent burnout.
The task of the occupational physician is to preserve health in the workplace, whether in terms of physical or mental health. There are two ways of doing this: firstly, **through collective** surveillance in the workplace to identify any malfunctions in the organisation and working conditions, and secondly, through **individual** monitoring of workers.
By establishing a link between health and work, it will be able to recommend appropriate means of prevention [15].
Like most authors, and in line with the preventive approach followed in occupational medicine, we will approach prevention in terms of collective and individual prevention.

1.11.1 Collective prevention

1.11.1.1 Working environment

For Maslach and his team, the causes lie mainly in the work environment, but most research has focused more on individual strategies[113], as they tend to be less costly (at least immediately), than interventions which target change at an organisational level[111].
It is essential to put in place preventive measures aimed at eliminating or reducing the factors responsible for burnout:

- Plan the work, assess the workload and try to reduce demands where they are too great, or provide the resources needed to meet them.
- Define more precise work objectives and determine each person's level of responsibility in order to remove any role ambiguities[15].
- Giving more decision-making power, which helps to mitigate the negative effects of work overload [114].
- Ensuring cohesion and harmonious relations within the team.
- Encouraging social support: support plays a central role, and is the factor most regularly identified as a determining factor.

Professional support is part of social support and has a moderating effect on the relationship between perceived stress and burnout [15], particularly if it is provided by hierarchical superiors [115].

- Valuing skills and recognising knowledge gained through experience, whatever the job.
- Improving communication.
- Involve staff in decision-making as much as possible.
- Increasing control and autonomy.

Indeed, autonomy at work considerably reduces burnout [114].

- To promote a working environment where effort, equity and fairness are recognised.

1.11.1.2 Training

Staff training helps maintain enthusiasm for the job and the acquisition of new knowledge.

1.11.2 Individual prevention

1.11.2.1 Stress management

- Helping the individual to cope with work-related stressors, using coping strategies.
- Adopt a more balanced lifestyle, take part in sporting activities, have hobbies and develop outside work[65].
- Implement relaxation techniques [25].

Relaxation is a physiological response that antagonises the stress response. It plays an important role in preventing burnout[15].

1.11.2.2 Psychotherapeutic care

Individual burnout therapy must focus on at least two aspects: the first concerns the "chronic stress" dimension and the second targets more specifically the relationship with others and the area of self-assertion[25] .

1.11.2.3 Treatment

If the burnout syndrome is severe, two to three months' sick leave may be necessary, with a prescription for a moderate dose of antidepressants (combined with psychotherapy is recommended)[35].

1.11.3 Preventing burnout in doctors

Given the scale of the burnout phenomenon and its seriousness among doctors, we are going to detail other preventive measures adapted to the medical environment.

1.11.3.1 Teaching

Include courses on burnout in university curricula (which are also taught to paramedics). Teach future doctors that they cannot cure all patients, that they are not all-powerful, and how they should behave towards patients (doctor-patient relationship).

1.11.3.2 Continuing medical education

It is essential for doctors to take part in continuing medical education, to keep their knowledge up to date.

Themes such as dealing with suffering, illness, death, end-of-life support, dealing with violence, etc. must also be addressed.

They need to be constantly informed and made aware of burnout syndrome.

1.11.3.3 Ensuring a good working environment

A non-secure environment is stressful. The presence of security guards or other people who can act in the event of violence will have a reassuring effect[115].The workload should be distributed evenly between doctors.

Support, recognition and appreciation are essential, especially from line managers.

Preventing burnout, which is the responsibility of all doctors, healthcare systems and the organisations in which they practise, involves promoting the well-being of doctors [116].

1.11.3.4 Taking care of yourself to better take care of others

Listen to yourself so that you can treat others well, avoid self-prescribing and have a doctor who is preferably neither a friend nor a relative, work on helping others because caring for others is not an easy task, don't hesitate to ask for help when you need it, etc. [15].

1.11.3.5 Setting up discussion groups in departments

Doctors are wary of talking groups, because they risk awakening suffering that is hidden and ignored by the doctors themselves [98].

This discussion group will enable team members to get together within the department, to communicate and express themselves about their work and to value it, in order to transform the suffering they feel into pleasure[15].

It is important to stress the importance of expression and exchange, which provide an opportunity to share the difficulties faced by everyone and, above all, to break out of isolation[65].

1.11.3.6 Balint groups

The Balint groups were introduced in England by the Hungarian doctor, psychologist and psychoanalyst Michael Balint[37].

This group is made up of doctors or other healthcare professionals with a maximum of 15 participants; it is led by a psychoanalyst, a psychiatrist and/or another doctor with good experience of the Balint group[117]; the aim of these training courses is to work on "the psychological and relational dimensions of the practice of the medical professions"[118].

Balint popularised and disseminated within the medical profession the idea that it was the doctor himself who had a predominant role in the treatment of illness. He made doctors aware of the dynamic relationship between doctor and patient [15].
Taking part in this group is an interesting way of getting to know yourself and developing your emotional potential.
The role of the group leader is very important, so that all attention is focused on the doctor-patient relationship and the doctor's personal problems are avoided [117].

1.11.4 Conclusion

If we want to put a stop to demotivation in the medical profession, we need to take action on both internal and external factors [98].

- Internal factors: acting on the individual (using psychiatric and psychoanalytical approaches, etc.), acting on systems (using sociological and environmental approaches, stress factors, etc.) and acting on the professional ideal (using a guilt-free approach, personality type, , etc.).
- External factors: urgently implement institutional, ministerial and other measures...

PRACTICAL PART

II. OBJECTIVES OF THE STUDY

Main objective

Assessing the prevalence of burnout syndrome in a population of general practitioners in the Wilaya of Sétif

Secondary objectives

- Estimate the score for the three dimensions of burnout: emotional exhaustion, depersonalisation and personal fulfilment.
- Determining the factors predisposing to burnout syndrome (BO).
- Identifying the consequences of burnout.
- Suggest preventive measures.

III. FRAMEWORK OF THE STUDY

III.1 GEOGRAPHICAL DATA FOR THE WILAYA OF SETIF

The wilaya of Sétif, the capital of the high plateaux, covers an area of 6,549.64 km^2, rises to an altitude of 1,100 m and is located in eastern Algeria. The total population of the wilaya is estimated at 1,489,979 (Recensement Général de la Population et de l'Habitat: RGPH 2008). It is 300km from the capital (Algiers) and borders the following wilayas: Jijel and Bejaï'a to the north, Mila to the east, Bordj-Bou-Arreridj to the west and the wilayas of Batna and M'sila to the south. Administratively, the wilaya of Sétif is made up of 20 daifas divided into 60 communes. (Appendix 2)

III.2 HEALTH INFRASTRUCTURE

The wilaya of Sétif has 10 hospitals and 9 EPSP with 68 polyclinics and 230 treatment rooms (appendix 2). The total number of GPs practising in these facilities on 31 March 2015 was 813 (DSP data for 2015).

IV. METHODS

IV.1 TYPE AND PERIOD OF THE STUDY

This is a cross-sectional survey conducted over a period from December 2016 to December 2017.

IV .2 TARGET POPULATION

The target population is represented by general practitioners practising in the public sector in the wilaya of Sétif at the CHU, EPSP, EPH, EHS and EH, whose total workforce was 813 in 2016 (data from the DSP and the CHU).

V V.3 STUDY POPULATION

Our study population consists of a representative sample of 463 general practitioners practising in the public sector in the 60 communes of the Wilaya of Sétif.

VI .3.1 Inclusion criteria

All GPs on the nominative list drawn at random during sampling.

VII 3.2 Non-inclusion criteria

- GPs with less than one year's experience.
- GPs on the list who have retired.
- GPs who were on long-term sick leave at the time of the survey.
- Two GPs who refused to reply to the questionnaire

In these cases, the GPs were replaced by those whose names followed immediately after them in the list.

IV.3.3 Sampling methods

The survey covered all 60 communes in the Wilaya of Sétif.

Sampling was based on stratified sampling, with the population stratified according to 4 health structures: EPSP, EHS, EPH+EH and CHU.
At each health facility, the subjects questioned were chosen at random from the nominative list.

IV.4 DATA COLLECTION

The data were collected using an anonymous questionnaire that we developed and which consists of two parts:

The first part dealt with (appendix 3)**:**

- Socio-demographic data
- Age
- Gender
- Marital status
- Number of children and dependants
- Chronic medical condition(s)
- Professional characteristics
- Place of work
- Working area
- Number of years in service
- Problems getting to work
- Late for work
- Average number of hours worked per week
- Night shifts
- Heavy workload
- Autonomy in decision-making at work
- Victim of physical or verbal aggression
- Feeling of injustice
- Quality of teamwork
- Support when needed
- Salary satisfaction
- Medical training (continuing)
- The characteristics of privacy
- Activities outside work (cultural activities, sport, leisure, etc.)
- Family time
- Personal and/or family problems (marital, financial, school problems for children ....)
- The impact of professional activity
- Addictive behaviour (coffee, tobacco, alcohol, drugs and psychotropic substances)
- Average number of hours sleep per night
- Presence of sleep disorders
- Work stoppage(s)
- Presence of somatic complaints
- Medical error
- Studying medicine again
- Need to retrain (change jobs)
- Suicidal thoughts
- An introduction to burnout syndrome

The second part focused on :

The Maslach Burnout Inventory Test (MBI)[54], which was validated in French by Dion and Tessier[48]. It is the most widely used questionnaire in the world today[52] and is scientifically validated (there are three versions for different professions).

In our study, we used the MBI-HSS (Maslach Burnout Inventory Human Services), since it is the one reserved for healthcare professionals (appendix 4).

IV.5 CONDUCT OF THE SURVEY

A feasibility pre-survey was carried out among around twenty GPs to rectify certain questionnaire items and finalise the questionnaire.

The survey took place at each GP's place of work. We travelled (with my own means) to hospitals, polyclinics and wards in the Wilaya. Each questionnaire was filled in on the spot and took about 20 to 30 minutes.

IV.6 STATISTICAL TECHNIQUES USED

Data was entered using Excel 10 and statistical analysis was performed using IBM SPSS version 20 (Statistical Package for the Social Sciences).

The statistical methods used are[119] :

- Descriptive statistics techniques: tabular presentation, graphical presentation and reduction and position parameters (means, standard deviation and range).
- Statistical comparison tests: Pearson's KHI-squared test used to compare proportions or Fisher's exact test for small numbers. Significance threshold $p<0.0\ 5$.
- Binary logistic regression is a powerful multivariate analysis method for quantifying the association between a phenomenon under study and each of the factors influencing it, while taking account of the simultaneous effect of the other factors. It also makes it possible to control for possible confounding biases[120]. We performed binary logistic regression using two methods, top-down and bottom-up (likelihood ratio), and included the variables that were significantly associated ($p<0.05$) with the three dimensions of the BO in the univariate analysis. This statistical method enabled us to develop a model to determine the factors predicting the three dimensions of burnout (EE, DP and AP) in our GPs, as well as the associated risk of each factor. The value of $p<0.05$ was considered a significant threshold, with a confidence interval (CI) of 95%.

IV.7 ETHICAL CONSIDERATIONS

The questionnaires were anonymous and no names appeared on them.

All the GPs who responded to the questionnaire gave their consent.

V. RESULTS

V.1 CHARACTERISTICS OF THE POPULATION STUDIED

V.1.1 Socio-demographic characteristics of GPs

V.1.1.1 Gender:

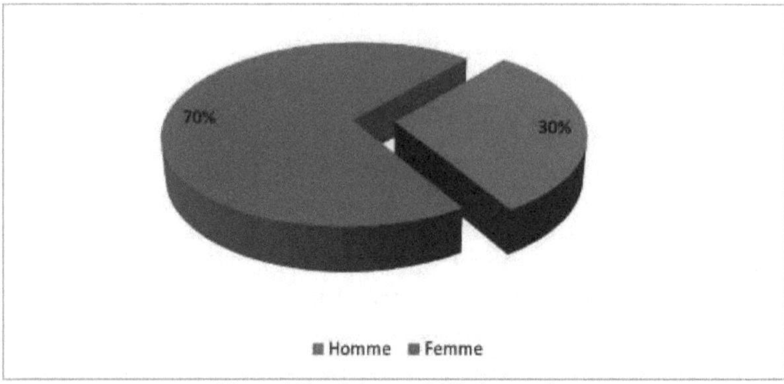

Figure 1 Breakdown of GPs by gender

Of the 463 doctors questioned, 324 (70%) were female and 139 (30%) male, giving a sex ratio of 0.42:1.

V.1.1.2 Age

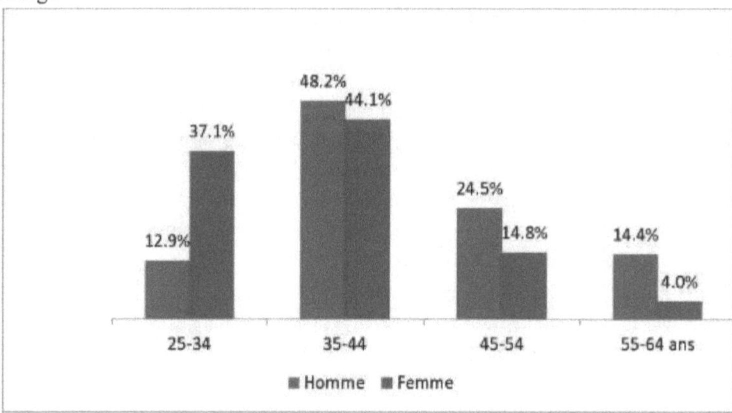

Figure 2 Distribution of GPs by age and gender

The average age of our population is 39 ± 8 years, ranging from 26 to 60. 75% are under 45.
Of the 324 female doctors, 81.2% are under 45.
Of the 139 male doctors, 61.1% were under 45.
There was a highly significant relationship between age and gender ($p<0.001$).

V.1.1.3 Marital status

	n	%
Single	78	16,9
Married	370	79,9
Divorced	13	2,8

Widowed	2	0,4
Total	463	100

Table 1 Breakdown of GPs by marital status

The majority (79.9%) of GPs are married.

V.1.1.4 Doctor's spouse

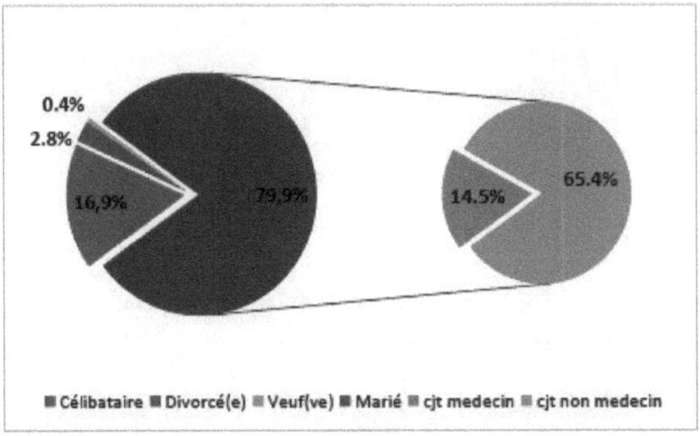

Figure 3 Distribution of GPs by marital status and spouse

Of the 370 (79.9%) married doctors, 67 (14.5%) have a doctor as a spouse.

V.1.1.5 Number of children

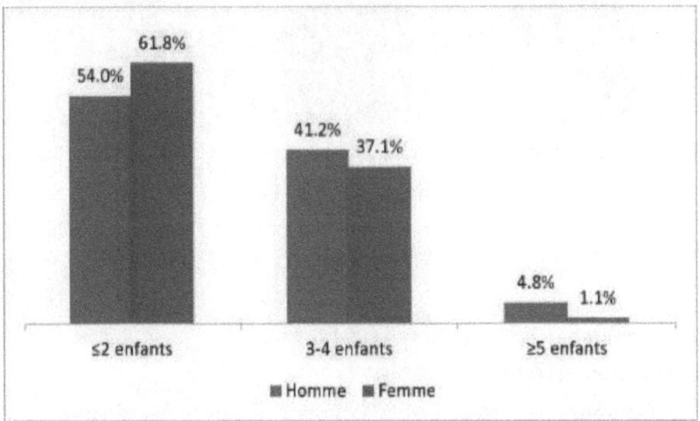

Figure 4 Distribution of GPs by number of children and gender

61.8% of women and 54% of men have 2 children or less.

Only 6% of the sample have 5 or more children. The average is 2 children ±1.

V.1.1.6 Number of dependants

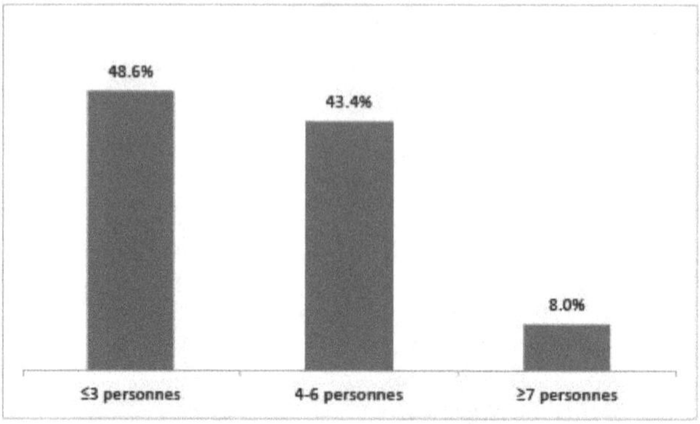

Figure 5 Distribution of GPs by number of dependants

17 (3.7%) doctors have no dependents, and 3 (0.6%) have 12 dependents (including children). Almost half (48.6%) have 3 or fewer dependants.

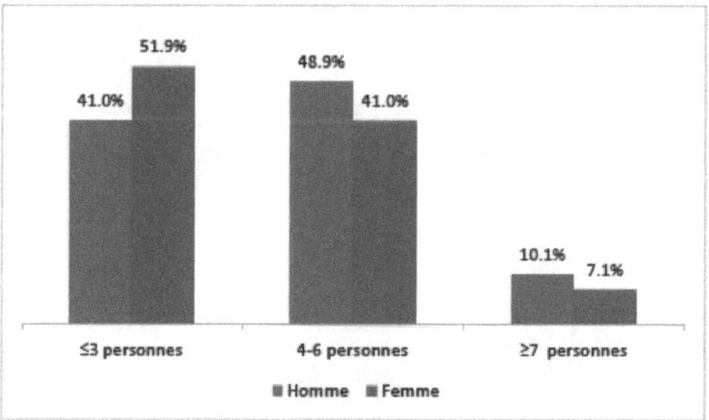

Figure 6 Distribution of GPs by number of dependants and gender

More than half of women have 3 or fewer dependants.
Men took on 4 to 6 people in 48.9% of cases.
V.1.1.7 Medical conditions

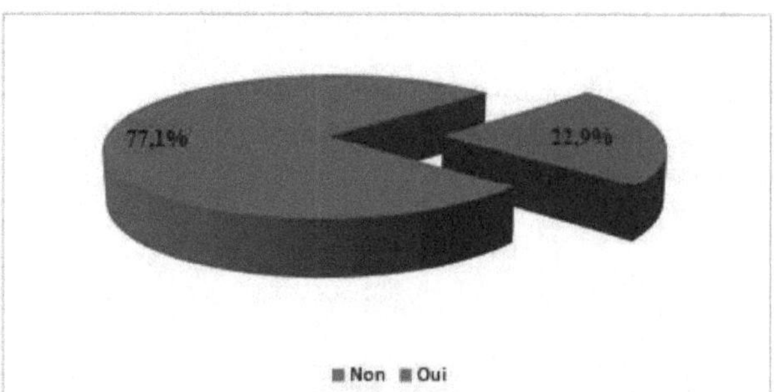

Figure 7 Distribution of GPs according to the presence of a medical condition

Of all GPs, 357 (77.1%) have no medical condition.

V.1.1.8 Type of medical condition

Medical conditions	n	%
HTA	30	6,5
Thyroid pathology	29	6,3
Diabetes	16	3,5
Psychiatric condition	10	2,1
Asthma	4	0,9
Other	40	8,6

Table 2 Breakdown of GPs by type of medical condition

Of the 106 (22.9%) doctors with a chronic pathology, 20 have 2 to 3 associated medical conditions.

Hypertension and thyroid disease come first, followed by diabetes.

V.1.1.9 Duration of the disease

		<5 years		5-10 years		>10 years	
	Workforce	n	%	n	%	n	%
HTA	30	18	60,0	7	23,3	5	16,7
Thyroid pathology	29	17	58,6	6	20,7	6	20,7
Diabetes	16	10	62,5	4	25,0	2	12,5
Psychiatric condition	10	4	40,0	1	10,0	5	50,0
Asthma	4	2	50,0	1	25,0	1	25,0
Other	40	15	37,5	15	37,5	10	25,0

Table 3 Distribution of GPs according to the duration of the pathology

More than half of hypertensives, diabetics and those with thyroid disease have had their condition for less than 5 years.

Of the 10 doctors with psychiatric conditions, half have had them for more than 10 years.

V.1.2 Characteristics of GPs' professional activity

V.1.2.1 Place of practice

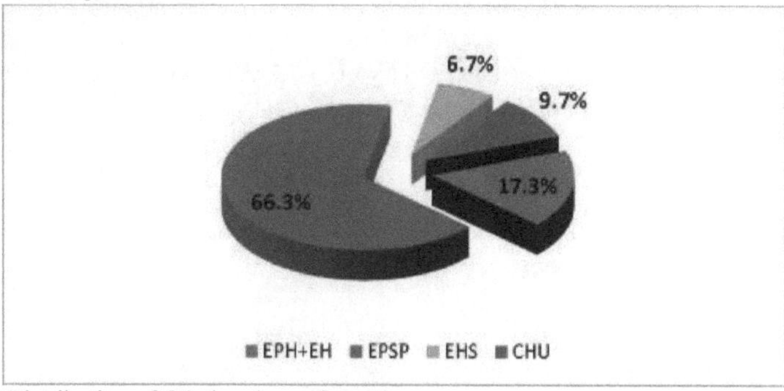

Figure 8 Distribution of GPs by place of practice

Two-thirds of GPs (66.3%) work in local public health establishments (EPSP), while only

6.7% work in specialist hospitals (EHS).

V.1.2.2 Working area

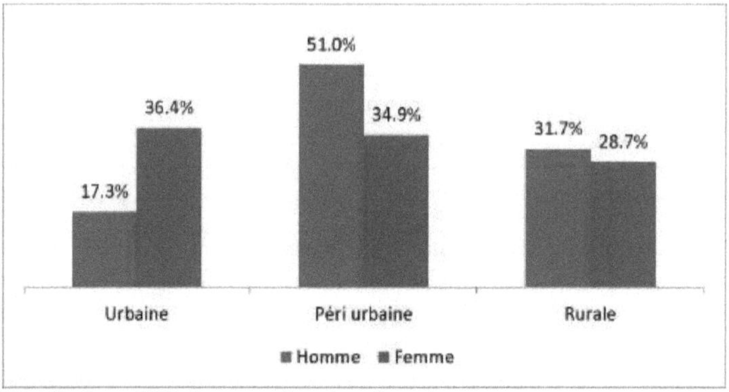

Figure 9 Distribution of GPs by area of work and gender

Female doctors worked mainly in urban (36.4%) and peri-urban (34.9%) areas, whereas male doctors worked in peri-urban (51%) and rural (31.7%) areas, with a highly significant relationship ($p<0.001$).

V.1.2.3 Number of years in service

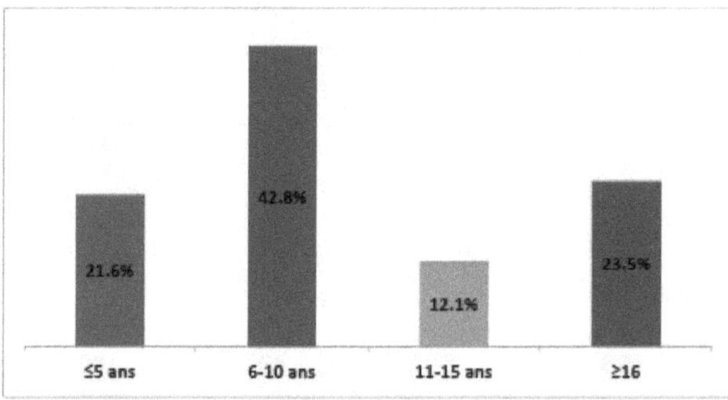

Figure 10 Breakdown of GPs by number of years in practice

The average number of years in practice was 11 years ± 7.7 years, with 4 doctors practising for 1 year (0.9%) and 1 doctor practising for 32 years (0.2%).

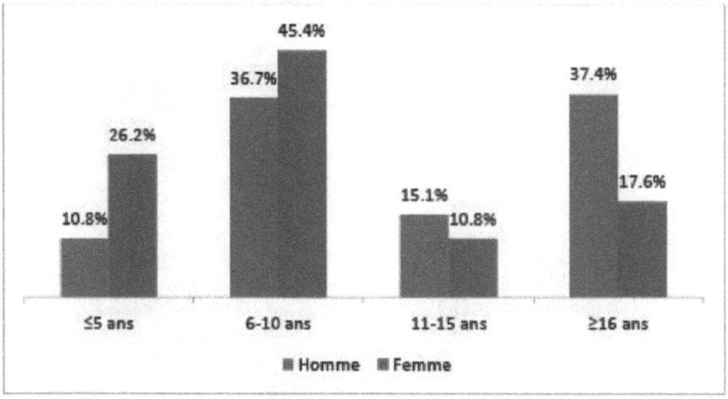

Figure 11 Distribution of GPs by number of years in practice and gender

71.6% of women have been working for 10 years or less. More than half (52.5%) of men have been in the profession for 11 years or more.
The relationship between number of years in practice and gender was highly significant ($p<0.001$).

V.1.2.4 Commuting problems

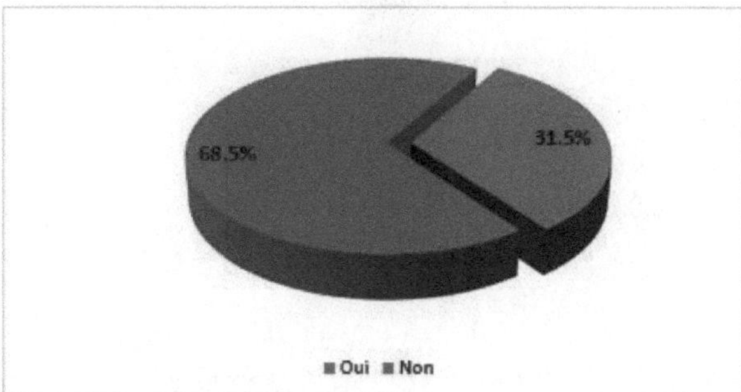

Figure 12 Distribution of GPs according to transport problems to work
work

68.5% of doctors do not complain about transport problems
V.1.2.5 Delayed work

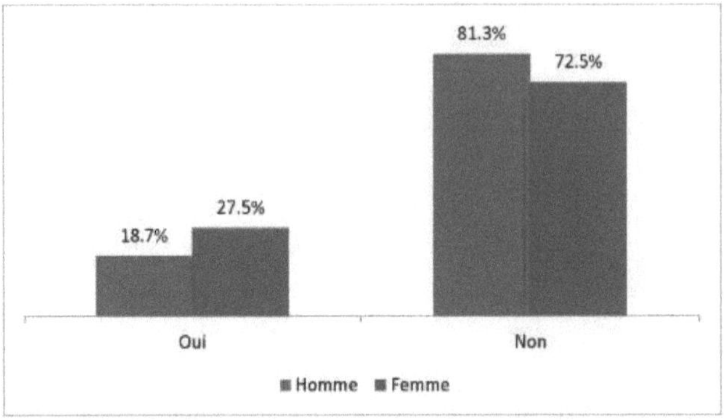

Figure 13 Distribution of GPs according to lateness to work and gender

27.5% of women admit to arriving late for work, compared with 18.7% of men.
The difference is significant ($P<0.05$).

V.1.2.6 Number of hours worked per week

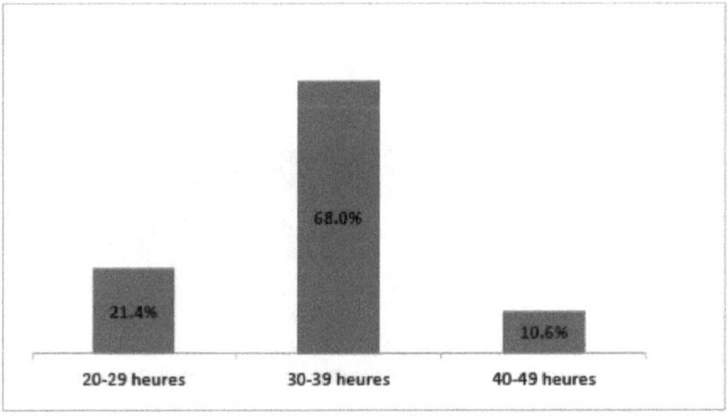

Figure 14 Distribution of GPs by number of hours worked per week

The average number of hours worked per week was 31.4 ± 5.4 hours, with a minimum of 20 hours for 22 (4.8%) doctors and a maximum of 45 hours for 4 (0.4%) of them. Over 2/3 (68%) of GPs work between 30 and 39 hours a week.

V.1.2.7 Working hours

	Frequency	%
Normal day	359	77,6
Day care	51	11,0
Night work	13	2,8
24-hour system	14	3,0
Other rhythms	26	5,6
Total	463	100

Table 4 Breakdown of GPs by work pattern

Of the 463 GPs, 77.6% work a normal day.
11% work day shifts, 3% work 24 hours and then rest for 3 days.

5.6% have other working patterns.

V.1.2.8 Night shifts

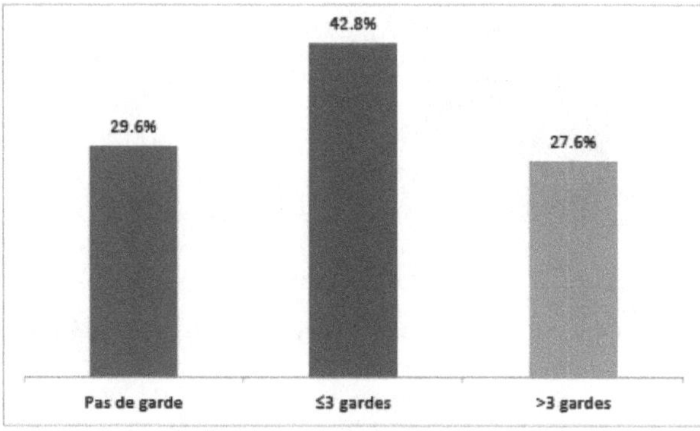

Figure 15 Distribution of GPs according to on-call duties

326 (70.4%) doctors do night shifts, and 198 (42.8%) do 1 to 3 shifts per month. The minimum number of shifts worked by doctors is one per month (5 doctors) and the maximum is 8 per month (2 doctors).

V.1.2.9 Workload

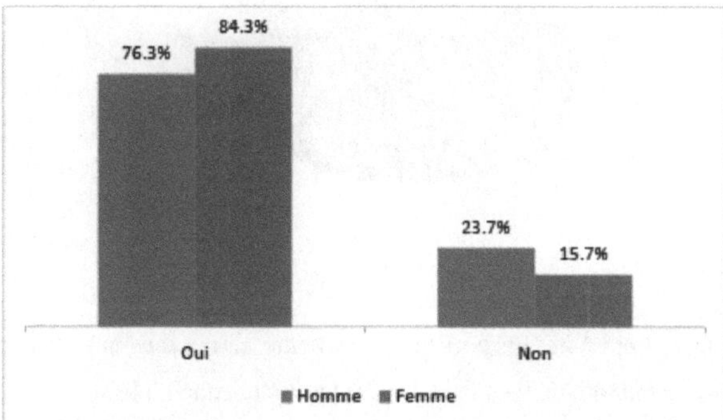

Figure 16 Breakdown of GPs by gender and workload

84.3% of female GPs versus 76.3% felt they had a heavy workload. The difference between the sexes is significant ($p<0.05$).

V.1.2.10Autonomy in decision-making

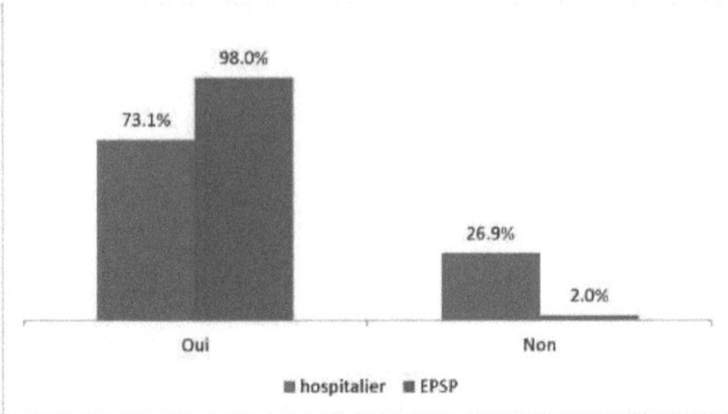

Figure 17 Distribution of GPs by place of practice and autonomy in decision-making

Almost all GPs (98%) practising in PHCs make decisions independently, whereas 26.9% of those practising in hospitals must first seek specialist advice, and the relationship is significant ($p<0.001$).

V.1.2.11 Attacks

V.1.2.11.1 Victims of assault

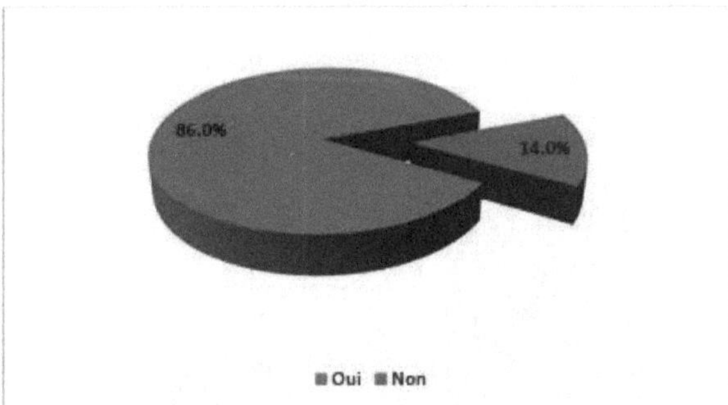

Figure 18 Distribution of GPs according to whether or not they have been attacked.

398 GPs, or 86%, stated that they had suffered at least one attack (physical or verbal) since they started practising.

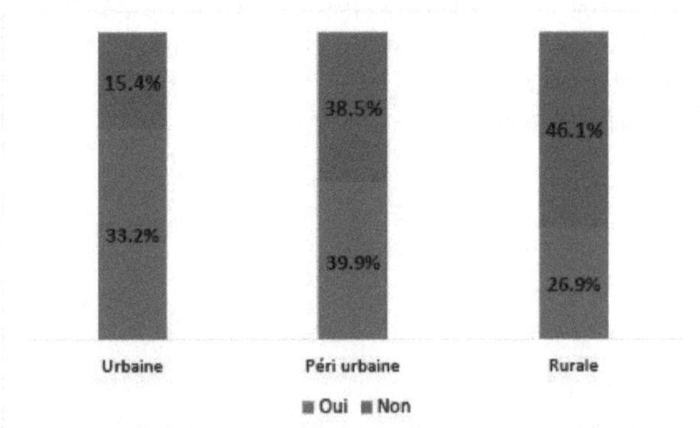

Figure 19 Distribution of GPs according to whether or not they have been attacked, by work

area

GPs suffer fewer assaults in rural areas (26.9%) than in other areas, and the link is significant ($p<0.01$).

V.1.2.11.2 Physical and verbal aggression

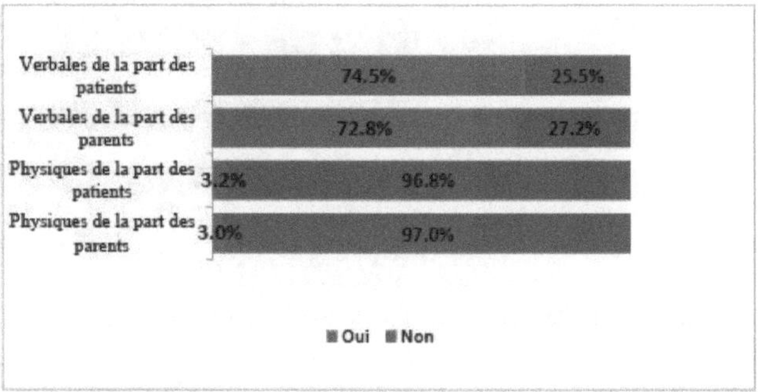

Figure 20 Distribution of GPs according to whether or not they have been physically or verbally assaulted

Of the 398 doctors who had been attacked, almost 3/4 (74.5%) had suffered at least one verbal attack from patients, and 72.8% from parents. As for physical aggression, doctors suffered almost the same frequency from patients (3.2%) and parents (3%).

V.1.2.12 Feeling of injustice

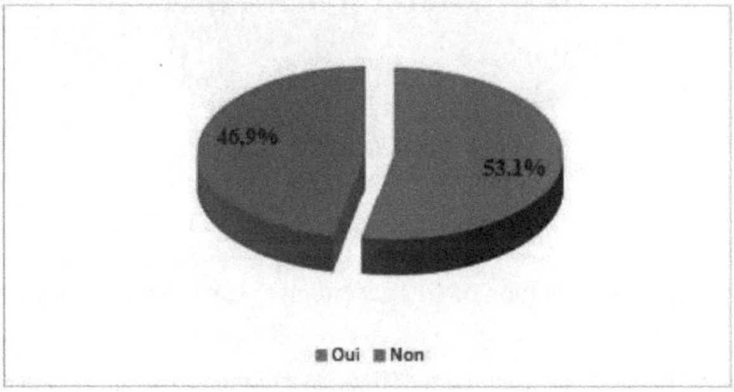

Figure 21 Distribution of GPs according to the existence of a feeling of injustice

More than half (246 or 53.1%) of GPs feel a sense of injustice in their workplace.

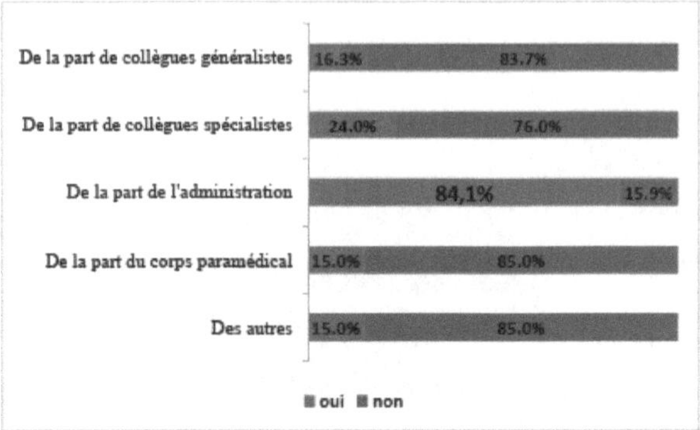

Figure 22 Distribution of GPs according to the origin of the feeling of injustice

Of the 246 doctors who said they felt a sense of injustice, 84.1% felt it from the administration.

V.1.2.13Quality of teamwork

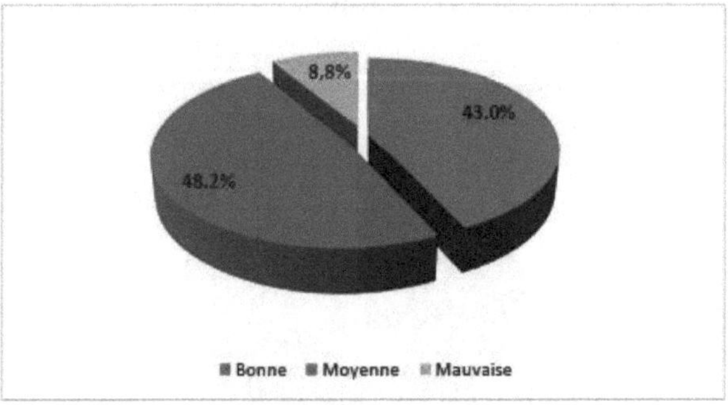

Figure 23 Distribution of GPs according to teamwork atmosphere

Almost half (48.2%) of GPs say that the working environment is average, and 8.8% consider it to be poor.

V.1.2.14 Support in case of need

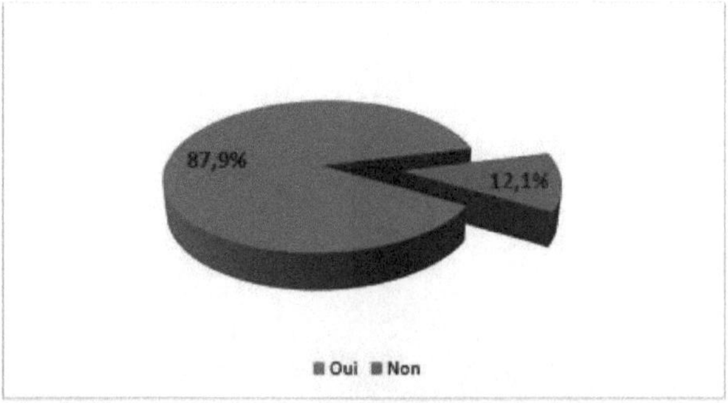

Figure 24 Distribution of GPs according to support in case of need

407 (87.9%) doctors say they receive support if they need it.

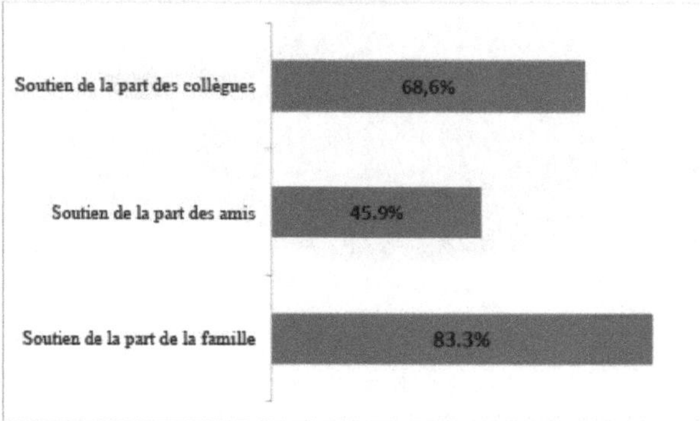

Figure 25 Distribution of GPs according to the different categories that support them

Of the 407 doctors who said they received support, 83.3% received it from their family.

V.1.2.15Salary

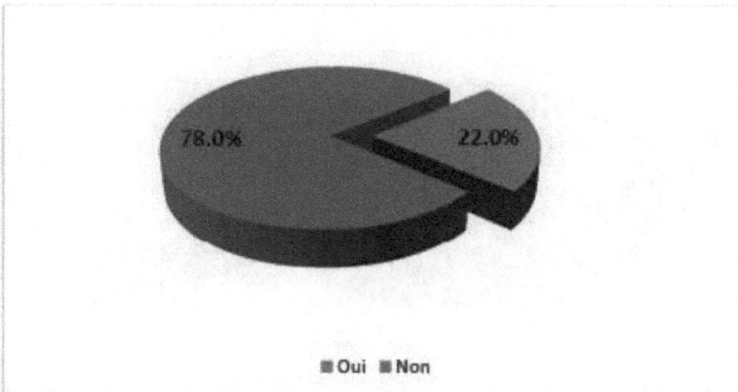

Figure 26 Distribution of GPs according to salary satisfaction

78% of GPs are not satisfied with their salary.

V.1.2.16Continuing medical education

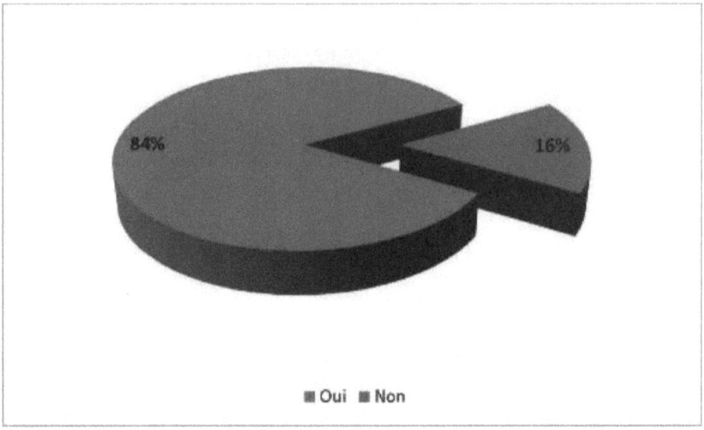

Figure 27 Distribution of GPs according to continuing medical education attendance

84% of GPs have taken part in continuing medical education.

V.1.2.17 The need for continuing medical education

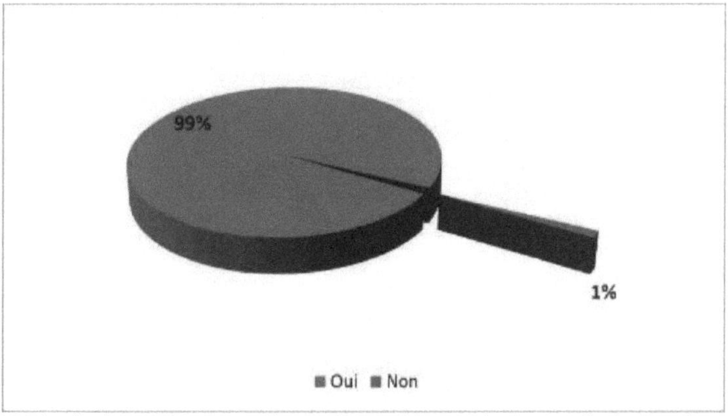

Figure 28 Distribution of GPs according to the need for continuing medical education

Almost all GPs (99%) recognise the need for and importance of continuing medical education.

V .1.3 Characteristics of privacy

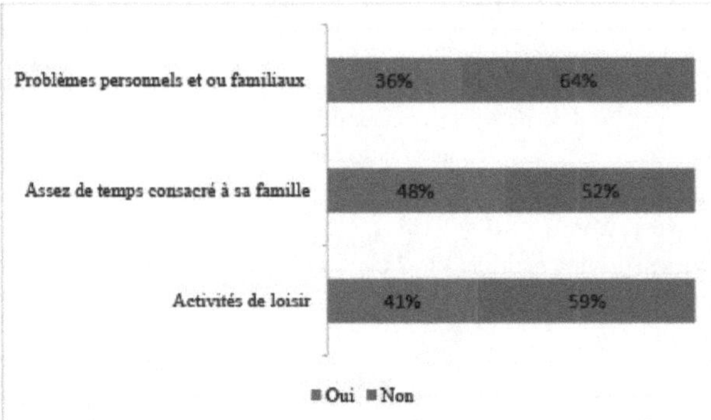

Figure 29 Breakdown of GPs by private life characteristics

64% of GPs say they have no personal or family problems.
More than half (52%) say they can't devote enough time to their family, and 59% say they don't have time for any activity outside work.

V .2 IMPACT OF PROFESSIONAL ACTIVITY ON THE POPULATION STUDIED

V .2.1 Addictions

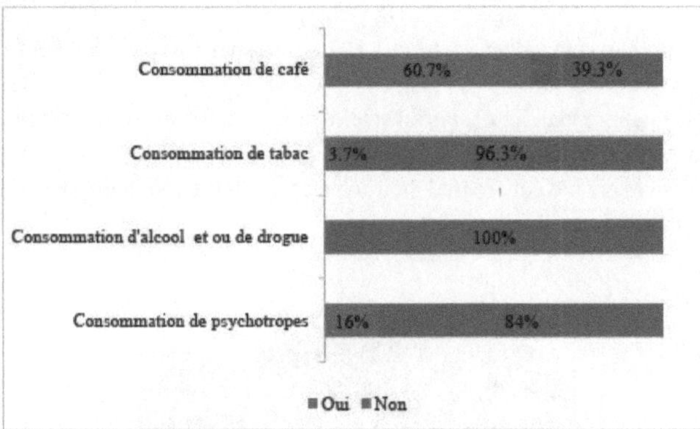

Figure 30 Distribution of GPs according to addictive behaviour

281 (60.7%) GPs drink coffee.
17 doctors, or 3.7%, are smokers, and all of them are male.
None of the doctors reported using alcohol or drugs.
16% of them have taken or are still taking psychotropic drugs.

V.2.1.1 Coffee

		Workforce	%	Total (%)
Number of cups / day	< 2	211	75,1	281 (100)
	> 2	70	24,9	
Duration (year)	<10	78	27,8	281 (100)
	10-20	150	53,4	

	>20	53	18,8	

Table 5 Distribution of MGs by number of cups of coffee per day and duration of consumption
consumption in years

Coffee consumption among the 281 GPs varied from 1 to 8 cups a day, and with a number of years from 1 to 40.
3/4 (75.1%) of these consumers drink 1 to 2 cups a day, and more than half (53.4%) for 10 to 20 years.

V.2.1.2 Tobacco

		Workforce	Percentage	Total (%)
Number of cigarettes / day	< 8	7	41,2	17 (100)
	> 8	10	58,8	
Duration (year)	< 15	8	47,1	17 (100)
	> 15	9	52,9	
Increase in tobacco consumption in the last 12 months	Yes	3	17,6	17 (100)
	No	14	82,4	

Table 6 Breakdown of GPs by number of cigarettes smoked per day and duration of smoking in years

The amount of tobacco smoked varies from 1 to 20 cigarettes a day, with the number of years smoked ranging from 3 to 35.
Of the 17 smokers, more than half (58.8%) smoked more than 8 cigarettes a day, and 52.9% had smoked for more than 15 years.
Only 3 (17.6%) smokers have increased their tobacco consumption in the last 12 months.

V.2.1.3 Psychotropic drugs

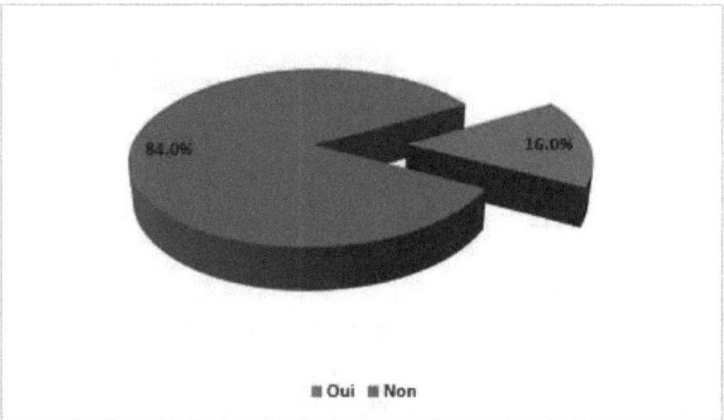

Figure 31 Breakdown of GPs by psychotropic drug use

16% of doctors use psychotropic drugs.

Psychotropic drugs	n	%
Self-medication	50	67,6
Medical prescription	24	32,4
< 5 years	40	54,1

> 5 years	34	45,9
Stop	31	41,9
Occasional use	20	27
Regular intake	23	31,1

Table 7 Breakdown of GPs who use psychotropic drugs

Of the 74 (16%) GPs who use psychotropic drugs, more than 2/3 (67.6%) self-medicate, with more than half (54.1%) taking them for less than 5 years.
58.1% of doctors who use psychotropic drugs do so occasionally or regularly.

V.2.2 Sleep

V.2.2.1 Nombre d'heures de sommeil par nuit

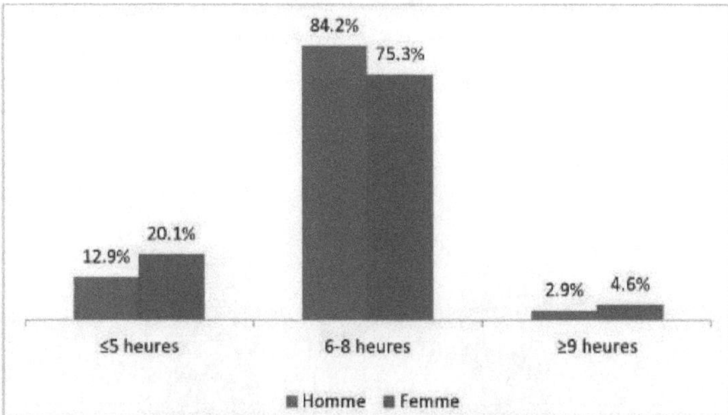

Figure 32 Distribution of GPs by sex and number of hours of sleep per night

The average number of hours of sleep per night in our population was 6.5 hours ± 1 hour, with a minimum of 2 hours (1 doctor) and a maximum ofll hours (2 doctors).
The majority of doctors sleep between 6 and 8 hours a night (75.3% for men vs. 84.2% for women), with no significant difference.

V.2.2.2 Sleep disorders

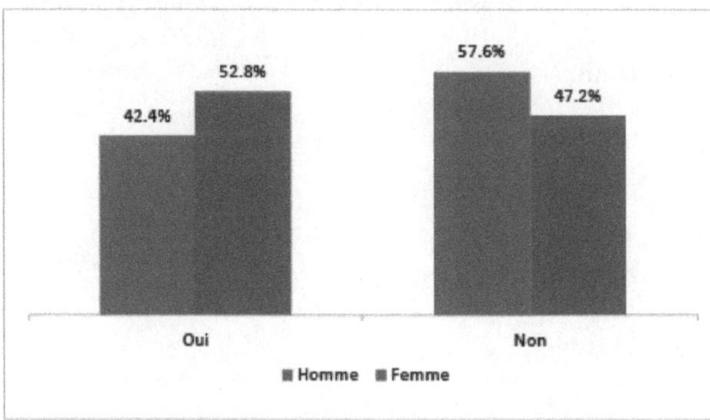

Figure 33 Breakdown of GPs by sex and sleep disorders

More than half of GPs who complain of sleep problems are female (52.8%), with a significant association (p<0.05).

V.2.3 Work stoppage(s)

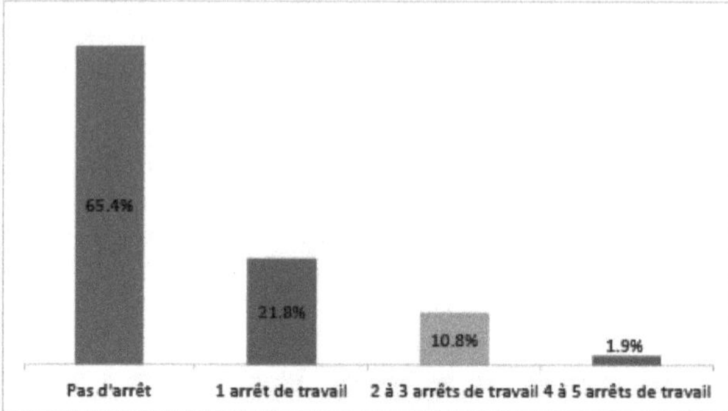

Figure 34 Distribution of GPs by number of work stoppages filed

65.4% of GPs had not filed any work stoppages and 1.9% had filed 4 or 5 stoppages in the 12 months preceding the questionnaire.

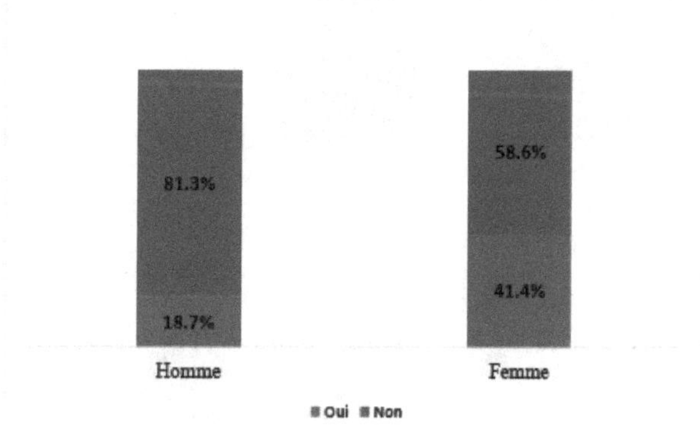

Figure 35 Distribution of GPs by number of days off work and gender

Of the GPs who filed a work stoppage, 41.4% were women, compared with 18.7% of men (p<0.001).

V.2.4 Somatic complaints

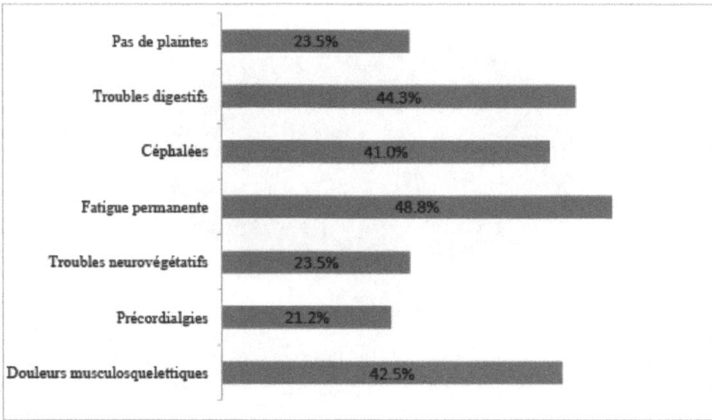

Figure 36 Breakdown of GPs by complaints reported

109 (23.5%) GPs had no somatic complaints.
354 (76.5%) of the doctors questioned reported the following somatic complaints:

- 48.8% complain of constant fatigue
- 44.3% digestive problems
- 42.5% musculoskeletal pain
- 41% headaches
- Then come in 5th and 6th place neurovegetative disorders (23.5%) and precordialgia (21.2%).

Of the doctors who complained, 21 (5.9%) reported all 6 complaints at the same time.

V.2.5 Fear of medical error

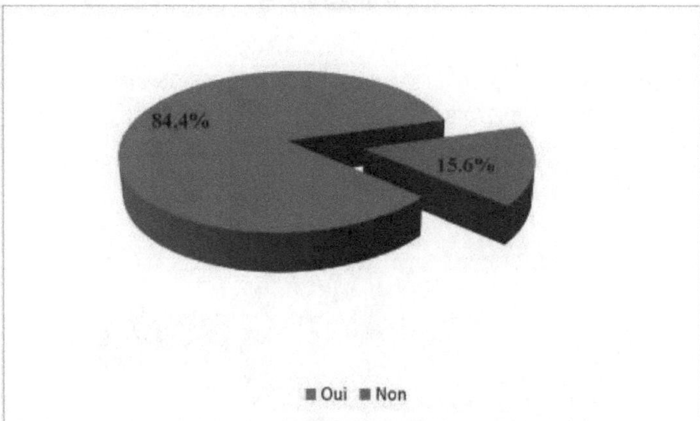

Figure 37 Répartition des MG selon la peur de commettre une erreur médicale

84.4% of doctors fear making a medical error.

V.2.6 Studying medicine again

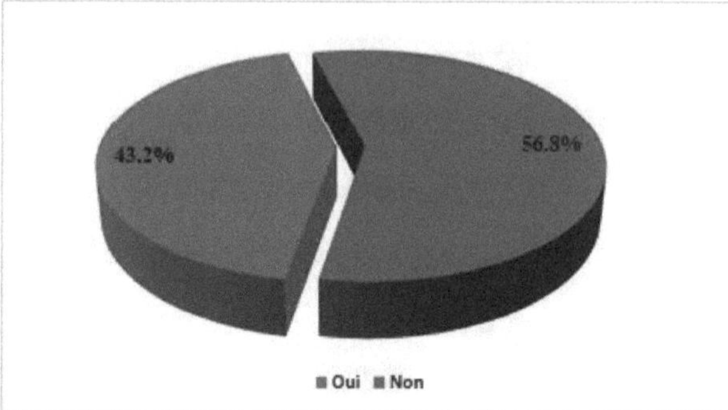

Figure 38 Distribution of GPs by desire to repeat medical studies

When doctors were asked whether they would choose to become a GP again in the same situation they would find themselves in if they had this choice, more than half (56.8%) replied in the negative.

V.2.7 Changer de métier

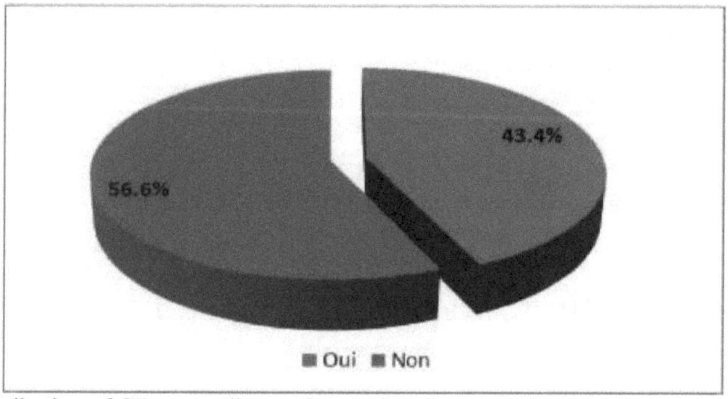

Figure 39 Distribution of GPs according to the need to change profession

43.4% of GPs feel the need to retrain.

V.2.8 Suicidal ideation

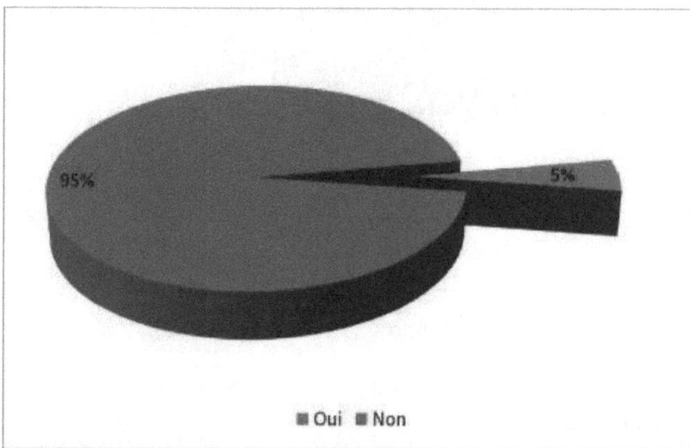

Figure 40 Distribution of GPs according to suicidal ideation

23 (5%) GPs had suicidal thoughts (3 males and 20 females).

V.2.9 Knowledge of Burnout

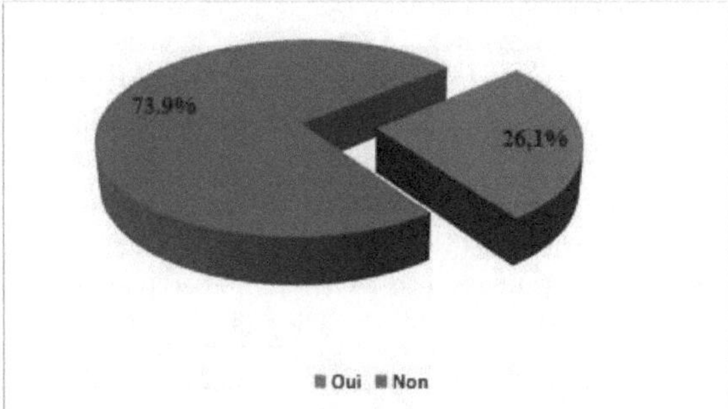

Figure 41 Distribution of GPs according to whether or not they have heard of the OB

73.9% of GPs have never heard of this syndrome.

V.3 EVALUATION OF THE BO DES MG

	High	Moderate	Bottom	Average score	Scope
	n (%)	n (%)	n (%)	± ET	
EE	**175 (37,8)**	169 (36,5)	119 (25,7)	26,12 ±12	0-54
DP	**57 (12,3)**	122 (26,3)	284 (61,3)	5,46 ± 5	0-24
AP	212 (45,8)	169 (36,5)	**82 (17,7)**	38,43 ± 5	22-48

(SD: Standard deviation)

Table 8 Distribution of GPs according to their level of burnout in each of the three dimensions

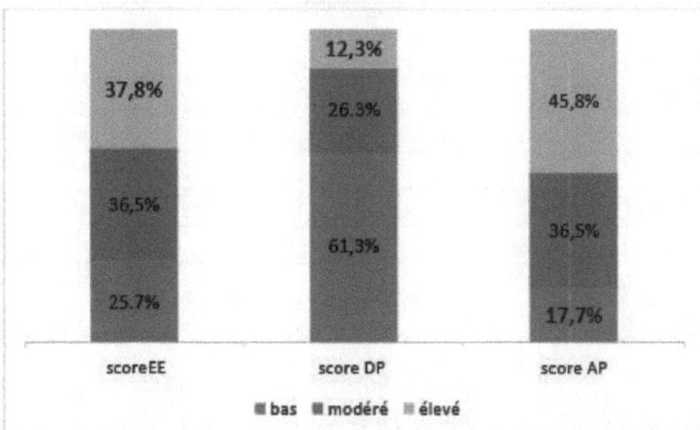

Figure 42 Distribution of GPs according to their level of burnout in each of the three dimensions

49% (227) of doctors were suffering from burnout, thus presenting at least one of the pathological dimensions.

175 doctors, or **37.8%,** had high emotional exhaustion, with an average score of 26.12 ±12, with extremes ranging from 0 to 54.

57 doctors (**12.3%**) had a high depersonalisation or dehumanisation syndrome, with an average score of 5.46 ± 5 and extremes ranging from 0 to 24.
Personal fulfilment was poor or low in **17.7%** of cases (82 GPs), with an average score of 38.43±5 and extremes ranging from 22 to 48.
15 doctors (3.2%) were in **severe BO**, i.e. they had a high level of burnout for all 3 components, while 74 doctors (**16%**) had none of the components of pathological burnout.
40 doctors, i.e. 8.6%, had two-dimensional burnout, i.e. both dimensions were affected (high EE and high PD)

V .4 FACTORS ASSOCIATED WITH BO

V .4.1 Factors associated with high EE

V .4.1.1 High emotional exhaustion and characteristics of the study population

V .4.1.1.1 High EE and socio-demographic characteristics

	Echantillons des MG		High EE MG		P
Variables	n	%	n	%	
Gender					>0,05
Men	139	30,0	45	32,4	
Woman	324	70,0	130	40,1	
Age (years)					>0,05
25-34	138	29,8	51	37,0	
35-44	210	45,4	84	40,0	
45-54	82	17,7	29	35,4	
55-64	33	7,1	11	33,3	
Marital status					>0,05
No spouse	93	20,1	43	46,2	
With spouse (Married)	370	79,9	132	35,7	
Doctor's spouse					>0,05
Yes	67	14,5	18	26,9	
No	303	65,4	114	37,6	
Number of **childrenb**					>0,05
< 2	228	49,2	87	38,2	
> 2	157	33,9	52	33,1	
Number of dependants					>0,05
<3	225	48,6	88	39,1	
>3	238	51,4	87	36,6	
Medical condition(s)					**<0,05**
Yes	106	22,9	52	49,1	
No	357	77,1	123	34,5	

Table 9 Breakdown of socio-demographic variables according to high EE

The total number of GPs for each variable is 463, with 175 doctors in high EE. **a** The total number of GPs is 370, or 79.9%, with 132 doctors in high EE.
[b] The total number of GPs is 385, or 83.1%, with 139 doctors in high EE.
High EE did not vary with gender, age, marital status, whether or not the patient had a doctor spouse, number of children or number of people in care (p> 0.05).
There is a significant link between the presence of a high EE and having a medical condition

($p<0.05$).

V.4.1.1.2 High EE and professional activity characteristics

	1'.chiniti	lon of GPs	High EE MG		P
Variables	n	%	n	%	
Place of work					<0,001
Hospital structure	156	33,7	64	41,0	
EPSP	307	66,3	111	36,2	
Working area					<0,001
Urban	142	30,7	72	50,7	
Peri-urban	184	39,7	66	35,9	
Rural	137	29,6	37	27,0	
Number of years in service (years)					>0,05
<5	100	21,6	35	35,0	
6-15	254	54,9	101	39,8	
>15	109	23,5	39	35,8	
Transport problems					>0,05
Yes	146	31,5	62	42,5	
No	317	68,5	113	35,6	
Late for work					<0,01
Yes	115	24,8	55	47,8	
No	348	75,2	120	34,5	
Number of hours worked per week					>0,05
20-29	99	21,4	35	35,4	
30-39	315	68,0	118	37,5	
40-49	49	10,6	22	44,9	
Heavy workload					<0,001
Yes	379	81,9	164	43,3	
No	84	18,1	11	13,1	
Autonomy in decision-making					<0,05
Yes	415	89,6	152	36,6	
No	48	10,4	23	47,9	

Table 9 Breakdown of professional activity characteristics according to high EE

High EE is observed :

- In 41% of cases, they work in hospitals, compared with 36.2% at the EPSP level.
- In 50.7% of cases working in urban areas vs. 27% of those working in rural areas.
- In 43.3% of doctors who perceive their workload as very heavy. The influence of these parameters on emotional exhaustion is highly significant ($p<0.001$).

Arriving late or not being autonomous in decision-making at work are also significantly linked to high EE.

High EE and characteristics of professional activity (continued)

	Sample	on of GPs	High EE MG		P
Variables	n	%	n	%	
Victim of assault					<0,001
Yes	398	86,0	167	42,0	

No	65	14,0	8	12,3	
Feeling of injustice					<0,001
Yes	246	53,1	126	51,2	
No	217	46,9	49	22,6	
Quality of teamwork					<0,001
Good	199	43,0	50	25,1	
Average	223	48,2	97	43,5	
Wrong	41	8,8	28	68,3	
Support when needed					>0,05
Yes	407	87,9	150	36,9	
No	56	12,1	25	44,6	
Continuing medical education					>0,05
Yes	387	83,6	147	38,0	
No	76	16,4	28	36,8	

Table 10 Distribution of professional activity characteristics according to high EE (continued)

Being attacked or feeling unfair were significantly associated with high emotional exhaustion in 42% and 51.2% of cases respectively (p<0.001).
Working in a poor working environment is also linked to EE in 68.3% of cases, compared with 25.1% when the environment is good (p<0.001).
Not being supported resulted in a high EE in 44.6% of cases compared with 36.9% in the case of support, but this difference was not significant (p >0.05).
There was no significant relationship between attendance or non-attendance at medical training courses.

V.4.1.3 High EE and privacy characteristics

	Sample of GPs		High EE MG		.P
Variables	n	%	n	%	
Activity outside work					>0,05
Yes	188	40,6	67	35,6	
No	275	59,4	108	39,3	
Family time					<0,001
Yes	222	47,9	68	30,6	
No	241	52,1	107	44,4	
Personal and/or family problems					<0,001
Yes	168	36,3	83	49,4	
No	295	63,7	92	31,2	

Table 11 Breakdown of private life characteristics in function of high EE

- Feeling that you don't spend enough time with your family is linked to EE in 44.4% of cases.
- The existence of personal or family problems was observed in 49.4% of cases.

The influence of these two variables on EE was highly significant (p<0.001).

- The absence of leisure activities or activities outside work led to EE in 39.3% of cases, but there was no significant link.

V.4.1.2 High EE and impact of professional activity on the population studied

	Sample of GPs		High EE MG		P
Variables	n	%	n	%	
Café					>0,05
Yes	281	60,7	103	36,7	
No	182	39,3	72	39,6	
Tobacco					>0,05
Yes	17	3,7	3	17,6	
No	446	96,3	172	38,6	
Psychotropic drugs					**<0,001**
Yes	74	16,0	44	59,5	
No	389	84,0	131	33,7	

Table 12 Breakdown of addictive behaviours according to high EE

No link was observed between high emotional exhaustion and coffee or tobacco consumption. GPs who were exhausted consumed psychotropic drugs to a very high degree in 59.5% of cases ($p<0.001$).

High EE and impact on professional activity (continued!)

	Sample of GPs		High EE MG		P
Variables	n	%	n	%	
Number of hours sleep/night					>0,05
<6	224	48,4	96	42,9	
> 6	239	51,6	79	33,1	
Sleep disorders					**<0,001**
Yes	230	49,7	113	49,1	
No	233	50,3	62	26,6	
Time off work in the last 12 months					>0,05
Yes	160	34,6	65	40,6	
No	303	65,4	110	36,3	
Somatic complaints					**<0,001**
Yes	354	76,5	159	44,9	
No	109	23,5	16	14,7	

Table 13 Breakdown of variables according to high EE

The number of hours of sleep per night and time off work have no influence on the EE dimension.

Half (49.1%) of GPs who complained of sleep problems were emotionally exhausted, with a highly significant link ($p<0.001$).

This difference is also very significant among those who report somatic complaints in 44.9% of cases.

High EE and impact of professional activity (continued2)

	Sample	.on of GPs	High EE MG		P
Variables	n	%	n	%	
Fear of committing a medical error					**<0,001**
Yes	391	84,4	161	41,2	

No	72	15,6	14	19,4	
Studying medicine again					**<0,001**
Yes	200	43,2	51	25,5	
No	263	56,8	124	47,1	
Need to retrain (change jobs)					**<0,001**
Yes	201	43,4	104	51,7	
No	262	56,6	71	27,1	
Suicidal thoughts					>0,05
Yes	23	5,0	14	60,9	
No	440	95,0	161	36,6	

Table 14 Distribution of different variables according to high EE

There is a highly significant relationship between the first burnout dimension and the following variables:

- fear of committing a medical error (41.2%).
- not to study medicine again (47.1%).
- the desire to retrain (51.7%).

The link with suicidal thoughts was not found (p>0.05).

V.4.2 Factors associated with high PD

V.4.2.1 High PD and characteristics of the population studied

V.4.2.1.1 High PD and socio-demographic characteristics

	Sample of GPs		High DP MG		
Variables	n	%	n	%	P
Gender					>0,05
Men	139	30,0	17	12,2	
Woman	324	70,0	40	12,3	
Age (years)					>0,05
25-34	138	29,8	13	9,4	
35-44	210	45,4	33	15,7	
45-54	82	17,7	9	11,0	
55-64	33	7,1	2	6,1	
Marital status					>0,05
No spouse	93	20,1	14	15,1	
With spouse (Married)	370	79,9	43	11,6	
Spouse doctor					>0,05
Yes	67	14,5	9	13,4	
No	303	65,4	34	11,2	
Number of children					**<0,05**
< 2	228	49,2	32	14,0	
> 2	157	33,9	14	8,9	
Number of dependants					>0,05
<3	225	48,6	30	13,3	
>3	238	51,4	27	11,3	
Medical condition(s)					>0,05

Yes	106	22,9	12	11,3	
No	357	77,1	45	12,6	

Table 15 Breakdown of variations)socio-demographics as a function of high PD

Gender, age, family situation, having a doctor spouse, looking after family members financially or medically or having a medical condition have no influence on doctors' depersonalisation (p>0.05).

Having two or fewer children was significantly associated with depersonalisation in 14% of cases (p<0.05).

V.4.2.1.2 High PD and professional activity characteristics

	Sample of GPs		High DP MG		P
Variables	n	%	n	%	
Place of work					**<0,05**
Hospital structure	156	33,7	28	17,9	
EPSP	307	66,3	29	9,4	
Working area					>0,05
Urban	142	30,7	25	17,6	
Peri-urban	184	39,7	21	11,4	
Rural	137	29,6	11	8,0	
Number of years in service					>0,05
<5	100	21,6	13	13,0	
6-15	254	54,9	34	13,4	
>15	109	23,5	10	9,2	
Transport problems					>0,05
Yes	146	31,5	19	13,0	
No	317	68,5	38	12,0	
Late for work					**<0,01**
Yes	115	24,8	22	19,1	
No	348	75,2	35	10,1	
Number of hours worked per week					>0,05
20-29	99	21,4	9	9,1	
30-39	315	68,0	40	12,7	
40-49	49	10,6	8	16,3	
Heavy workload					**<0,01**
Yes	379	81,9	52	13,7	
No	84	18,1	5	6,0	
Autonomy in decision-making					>0,05
Yes	415	89,6	50	12,0	
No	48	10,4	7	14,6	

Table 16 Distribution of professional activity characteristics according to high PD

Doctors working in hospitals depersonalise their patients more than those working in PHCs (p<0.05).

Frequently arriving late and perceiving one's workload as heavy are also significantly linked to this dimension in 19.1% and 13.7% respectively.

No relationship was observed for the other variables.

High PD and characteristics of professional activity (continued)

	Sample of GPs		High DP MG		P
Variables	n	%	n	%	
Victim of assault					**<0,001**
Yes	398	86,0	55	13,8	
No	65	14,0	2	3,1	
Feeling of injustice					**<0,05**
Yes	246	53,1	38	15,4	
No	217	46,9	19	8,8	
Quality of teamwork					**<0,01**
Good	199	43,0	15	7,5	
Average	223	48,2	33	14,8	
Wrong	41	8,8	9	22,0	
Support when needed					0,05
Yes	407	87,9	50	12,3	
No	56	12,1	7	12,5	
Continuing medical education					>0,05
Yes	387	83,6	51	13,2	
No	76	16,4	6	7,9	

Table 17 Breakdown of job characteristics by high PD (continued)

Aggression had a very significant effect on depersonalisation (p<0.001).

A bad working environment depersonalises 22% of employees, compared with 7.5% when it is good, and this in a positive way.

Feeling unfairly treated was also linked to this dimension in 15.4% of cases.

V.4.2.1.3 High PD and privacy characteristics

	Sample of GPs		High DP MG		P
Variables	n	%	n	%	
Activity outside work					>0,05
Yes	188	40,6	23	12,2	
No	275	59,4	34	12,4	
Family time					**<0,001**
Yes	222	47,9	16	7,2	
No	241	52,1	41	17,0	
Personal and/or family problems					**<0,01**
Yes	168	36,3	32	19,0	
No	295	63,7	25	8,5	

Table 18 Breakdown of private life characteristics according to high PD

GPs who significantly depersonalise their patients :

- don't spend enough time with their families in 17% of cases.
- have personal or family problems in 19% of cases.

V.4.2.2 High PD and impact of professional activity on the population studied

	Sample of GPs		MG in	High PD	P
Variables	n	%	n	%	
Café					>0,05
Yes	281	60,7	39	13,9	
No	182	39,3	18	9,9	
Tobacco					>0,05
Yes	17	3,7	1	5,9	
No	446	96,3	56	12,6	
Psychotropic drugs					**<0,05**
Yes	74	16,0	16	21,6	
No	389	84,0	41	10,5	

Table 19 Breakdown of addictive behaviours according to high PD

The use of psychotropic drugs was significantly linked to this dimension in 21.6% of cases ($p<0.05$).

High PD and impact of professional activity on the population studied (suitel)

	Sample of GPs		High DP MG		P
Variables	n	%	n	%	
Number of hours sleep/night					>0,05
<6	224	48,4	28	12,5	
> 6	239	51,6	29	12,1	
Sleep disorders					**<0,01**
Yes	230	49,7	36	15,7	
No	233	50,3	21	9,0	
Time off work in the last 12 months					>0,05
Yes	160	34,6	21	13,1	
No	303	65,4	36	11,9	
Somatic complaints					**<0,001**
Yes	354	76,5	46	13,0	
No	109	23,5	11	10,1	

Table 20 Distribution of variables according to high PD

The number of hours of sleep per night has no influence on PD.

However, this dimension is significantly associated :

- sleep disorders in 15.7% of cases ($p<0.01$).
- the presence of somatic complaints in 13% of cases ($p<0.001$).

High PD and the impact of professional activity on the population studied (continued2)

	Sample of GPs		High DP MG		P
Variables	n	%	n	%	
Fear of committing a medical error					**<0,05**
Yes	391	84,4	52	13,3	
No	72	15,6	5	6,9	
Studying medicine again					**<0,05**
Yes	200	43,2	16	8,0	

No	263	56,8	41	15,6	
Need to retrain (change jobs)					<0,001
Yes	201	43,4	35	17,4	
No	262	56,6	22	8,4	
Suicidal thoughts					<0,05
Yes	23	5,0	7	30,4	
No	440	95	50	11,4	

Table 21 Distribution of different variables according to high PD

Doctors who significantly depersonalise their patients :

- are afraid of committing a medical error in 13.3% of cases.
- would not study medicine again in 15.6% of cases.
- would feel the need to retrain if they had the opportunity to do so in 17.4% of cases (p<0.001).
- had already had suicidal thoughts in 30.4% of cases.

V **.4.3 Factors associated with low PA**

V .4.3.1 Low PA and characteristics of the study population

V .4.3.1.1 Low PA and socio-demographic characteristics

	Sample of GPs		GP in low PA		
Variables	n	%	n	%	P
Gender					>0,05
Men	139	30	23	16,5	
Woman	324	70	59	18,2	
Age (years)					<0,01
25-34	138	29,8	33	23,9	
35-44	210	45,4	39	18,6	
45-54	82	17,7	7	8,5	
55-64	33	7,1	3	9,1	
Marital status					>0,05
No spouse	93	20,1	21	22,6	
With spouse (Married)	370	79,9	61	16,5	
Spouse doctor					>0,05
Yes	67	14,5	12	17,9	
No	303	65,4	49	16,2	
Number of children					<0,05
< 2	228	49,2	48	21,1	
> 2	157	33,9	16	10,2	
Number of dependants					>0,05
<3	225	48,6	48	21,3	
>3	238	51,4	34	14,3	
Medical condition(s)					>0,05
Yes	106	22,9	17	16,0	
No	357	77,1	65	18,2	

Table 22 Distribution of socio-demographic variables according to low PA

GPs under 35 have the lowest personal fulfilment (p<0.01).
Having fewer than two children means a significantly lower PA (p<0.05)
No significant relationship was observed between low PA and the other variables.
V.4.3.1.2 Low PA and professional activity characteristics

	Sample of GPs		GP in low PA		
Variables	n	%	n	%	P
Place of work					>0,05
Hospital structure	156	33,7	36	23,1	
EPSP	307	66,3	46	15,0	
Working area					>0,05
Urban	142	30,7	25	17,6	
Peri-urban	184	39,7	32	17,4	
Rural	137	29,6	25	18,2	
Number of years in service (years)					<0,01
<5	100	21,6	23	23,0	
6-15	254	54,9	48	18,9	
>15	109	23,5	11	10,1	
Transport problems					>0,05
Yes	146	31,5	26	17,8	
No	317	68,5	56	17,7	
Late for work					>0,05
Yes	115	24,8	23	20,0	
No	348	75,2	59	17,0	
Number of hours worked per week					>0,05
20-29	99	21,4	16	16,2	
30-39	315	68	56	17,8	
40-49	49	10,6	10	20,4	
Heavy workload					>0,05
Yes	379	81,9	68	17,9	
No	84	18,1	14	16,7	
Autonomy in decision-making					>0,05
Yes	415	89,6	71	17,1	
No	48	10,4	11	22,9	

Table 23 Distribution of professional activity characteristics according to low PA

During the first five years of a career, PA is significantly lower (p<0.01).
There is no significant link between this dimension of the BO and the other variables.
Low PA and characteristics of professional activity (continued)

	Sample of GPs		GP in low PA		
Variables	n	%	n	%	P
Victim of assault					<0,01
Yes	398	86	77	19,3	
No	65	14	5	7,7	

Feeling of injustice					>0,05
Yes	246	53,1	46	18,7	
No	217	46,9	36	16,6	
Quality of teamwork					**<0,05**
Good	199	43	30	15,1	
Average	223	48,2	46	20,6	
Wrong	41	8,8	6	14,6	
Support when needed					>0,05
Yes	407	87,9	69	17,0	
No	56	12,1	13	23,2	
Continuing medical education					**<0,05**
Yes	387	83,6	62	16,0	
No	76	16,4	20	26,3	

Table 24 Distribution of professional activity characteristics according to low PA (continued)

19.3% (p<0.01) of people who experienced aggression had low self-esteem.
Doctors who consider their working environment to be average have a significantly lower PA than those who consider it to be good or bad.
GPs who do not attend medical training courses have a significantly low PA in 26.3% of cases (p<0.05).
Feeling unfair or not being supported in times of need had no influence on this dimension (p>0.05).
V.4.3.1.3 Low AP and privacy characteristics

	Sample of GPs		GP in low PA		
Variables	n	%	n	%	P
Activity outside work					**<0,01**
Yes	188	40,6	25	13,3	
No	275	59,4	57	20,7	
Family time					**<0,05**
Yes	222	47,9	29	13,1	
No	241	52,1	53	22,0	
Personal and/or family problems					>0,05
Yes	168	36,3	38	22,6	
No	295	63,7	44	14,9	

Table 25 Breakdown of private life characteristics according to low PA

Low PA is significantly influenced by not having activities outside work (e.g. leisure) in 20.7% of cases, and not spending enough time with the family in 22%.
There was no link between the existence of personal or family problems and this dimension (p>0.05).
V.4.3.2 Low PA and impact of professional activity on the population studied

	Sample of GPs		GP in low PA		
Variables	n	%	n	%	P
Café					>0,05
Yes	281	60,7	45	16,0	

No	182	39,3	37	20,3	
Tobacco					>0,05
Yes	17	3,7	3	17,6	
No	446	96,3	79	17,7	
Psychotropic drugs					>0,05
Yes	74	16	17	23,0	
No	389	84	65	16,7	

Table 26 Breakdown of addictive behaviours according to low PA

Addictive behaviours do not influence this dimension of burnout (p>0.05).

Low PA and impact of professional activity on the population studied (suitel)

	Sample of GPs		GP in low PA		
Variables	n	%	n	%	P
Number of hours sleep / night					>0,05
<6	224	48,4	34	15,2	
> 6	239	51,6	48	20,1	
Sleep disorders					**<0,05**
Yes	230	49,7	49	21,3	
No	233	50,3	33	14,2	
Work stoppage(s) during the last 12 months					>0,05
Yes	160	34,6	35	21,9	
No	303	65,4	47	15,5	
Somatic complaints					>0,05
Yes	354	76,5	69	19,5	
No	109	23,5	13	11,9	

Table 27 Distribution of variables according to low PA

The number of hours of sleep, time off work or somatic complaints did not influence the presence of low personal fulfilment (p>0.05).

In this study, sleep disorders were significantly associated with low PA (21.3%).

Low PA and the impact of professional activity on the population studied (continued2)

	Sample of GPs		GP in low PA		
Variables	n	%	n	%	P
Fear of committing a medical error					>0,05
Yes	391	84,4	75	19,2	
No	72	15,6	7	9,7	
Studying medicine again					**<0,001**
Yes	200	43,2	25	12,5	
No	263	56,8	57	21,7	
Need to retrain					**<0,001**
Yes	201	43,4	51	25,4	
No	262	56,6	31	11,8	
Suicidal thoughts					>0,05
Yes	23	5	7	30,4	

No	440	95	75	17,0	

Table 28 Distribution of different variables according to low PA

There is no significant link between low PA and :
- the fear of committing a medical error.
- suicidal thoughts.

Doctors who do not want to study medicine again and who feel the need to change profession have a significantly lower PA ($p<0.001$).

V.5 MULTIVARIATE ANALYSIS

We performed binary logistic regression analyses to select the independent variables predictive of burnout in its three dimensions: EE, DP and AP.

V.5.1 High emotional exhaustion and associated factors

The classification table showed that the prediction, based on the most frequent category, enabled 83.4% of GPs participating in the study to be correctly classified.

Factors associated with high EE	OR (95% CI)	P
■ Heavy workload	4,50 (2,07 - 9,73)	0,0001
■ Somatic complaints	2,88 (1,47 - 5,67)	0,002
■ Fear of committing a medical error	2,37 (1,15 - 4,87)	0,019
■ Psychotropic drugs	2,33 (1,24 - 4,37)	0,009
■ Urban working area	2,24 (1,19 - 4,25)	0,013
■ Feeling of injustice	2,14 (1,35 - 3,41)	0,001
■ Place of practice: hospital structure	0,54 (0,32 - 0,90)	0,018
■ Studying medicine again	0,51 (0,32 - 0,82)	0,005
■ Quality of teamwork: average	0,39 (0,17 - 0,90)	0,026
■ Quality of teamwork: good	0,20 (0,09 - 0,48)	0,0001

95% CI: 95% confidence interval; OR: Odds ratio

Table 29 Independent explanatory variables associated with the occurrence of EE

As we can see, the regression model retained 10 significant predictors of EE out of the 17 associated variables in univariate analysis. The model showed that GPs with a heavy workload, somatic complaints, fear of making a medical error, use of psychotropic drugs, working in an urban area and those who felt a sense of injustice were more likely to suffer emotional exhaustion. On the other hand, doctors who worked in a hospital setting, with a good team, and who stated that they did not want to repeat their studies at medicine were less likely to be emotionally exhausted. It should be noted that **heavy workload** was the variable most likely to explain high EE (OR= 4.5).

V.5.2 High depersonalisation and associated factors

With regard to depersonalisation, the model explains only 14.4% of the variance (in the feeling of depersonalisation).

Factors associated with PD	OR (95% CI)	P
■ Need to retrain	2,43 (1,25 - 4,73)	0,009
■ Late for work	2,29 (1,16 - 4,51)	0,017
■ Making time for your family	0,41 (0,20 - 0,84)	0,015
■ Good teamwork	0,24 (0,09 - 0,68)	0,007

95% CI: 95% confidence interval; OR: Odds ratio

Table 30 Independent explanatory variables associated with the occurrence of feelings of depersonalisation

According to the model, doctors who needed to retrain and who arrived late for work were more likely to develop a feeling of depersonalisation. On the other hand, this depersonalisation was less likely among GPs who did not devote enough time to their families or among those who worked in a team under good conditions. The other factors were no longer significant in the multivariate analysis.

V.5.3 Low personal achievement and associated factors

The model obtained explains 83.4% of the variance in personal fulfilment, which is considered very satisfactory, given the exploratory nature of this study.

Factors associated with low PA	**OR (95% CI)**	**P**
- Number of children < 2	2,45 (1,32 - 4,53)	0,004
- Need to retrain	2,60 (1,48 - 4,55)	0,001

95% CI: 95% confidence interval; OR: Odds ratio

Table 31 Independent explanatory variables associated with the occurrence of low low personal fulfilment

According to the model, it is highly likely that GPs who had fewer than two children and those who felt the need to retrain had a low PA.

VI. DISCUSSION

VI.1 CHARACTERISTICS OF THE POPULATION STUDIED

VI.1.1 Socio-demographic characteristics of GPs

In our study, more than 2/3 (70%) of GPs were women, which bears witness to the feminisation of the medical profession in our society. The same rate (70.2%) was found among resident doctors in Sidi Bel-Abbes [9]. In a French study of general medical interns, there was also a preponderance of women (62.6%) [121]. A study published in 2006 reported that feminisation was accelerating in France in the younger generations, and that women were in the majority in the under-34 age group and in equal numbers in the under-40 age group. This observation has also been described in Germany, Great Britain and the United States[122].

We also noted that 81.2% of our doctors under the age of 45 were women, compared with 61.1% men, with a highly significant link between gender and age ($p<0.001$).

Our population was young, with 75% aged under 45, with an average age of 39 ± 8 years, ranging from 26 to 60 years. In a study of GPs in France, the mean age was much higher: 46.4 ± 7.3 years (extremes: 28-70 years) [3], while another study of GPs in 12 European countries also found this high rate (45.4 ± 8.5 years) [123].

The majority (79.9%) of doctors were married, of whom only 14.5% had a doctor as a spouse. The average number of children was 2 ±1, with extremes ranging from 0 to 8. It should be noted that women had fewer children than men, but not significantly so. This could be explained by the fact that they are unable to reconcile work and a large family. This gender difference in the number of children was also observed among GPs in Luxembourg, and was statistically significant [37]. A study of American surgeons reported that women thought that bringing up children slowed down their professional careers [124]. Although the Algerian mentality is different from that of Westerners, it could be that our women feel the same way, but this aspect was not addressed in the questionnaire.

Only 3.7% of doctors had no dependents at all, the rest were living with or financially (or at least medically) supporting one or more dependents. Almost half had 3 or fewer dependants.

77.1% (357) of our population had no medical condition. 106 GPs had at least one chronic condition: 86 of them had a single medical condition and 20 had 2 or 3 associated conditions. These conditions were, in order, hypertension, thyroid disease, diabetes, psychiatric conditions, asthma and other conditions (neurological, rheumatological, dermatological, etc.) with no significant relationship between the sexes. According to some authors, patients expect doctors to be in good health, and if they happen to be ill, this should not be perceptible to them. However, any illness or suffering they may have inevitably influences the way they assume their role as carers [125].

VI.1.2 Characteristics of GPs' professional activity

Two-thirds of GPs (66.3%) worked in local public health establishments (EPSP), while the remaining 1/3 worked in hospitals.

In terms of working area, the number of male doctors practising in rural areas was greater than the number of female doctors, with a significant relationship ($p<0.001$).

Almost 3/4 (71.6%) of the women had been working for 10 years or less, while more than half (52.5%) of the men had been working for more than 10 years, with a significant relationship ($p<0.001$). This could be explained, as we observed above, by the feminisation of the profession in recent years.

More than 2/3 of our population did not complain about the transport problem. However, more than 1/4 (27.5%) of the women admitted to arriving late for work, with a significant link between the sexes ($p<0.05$). The women said that they had to attend to their family obligations, especially looking after their children in the morning before going to work.
Around 9/10 (89.4%) of our sample worked less than 40 hours a week.
77.6% had a normal work pattern, i.e. they did not work alternating shifts, as is the case with other work patterns. The 326 doctors who worked night shifts averaged 3.5 ± 1 shifts per month.
The 137 doctors (29.6%) did not work night shifts for several reasons: -certain work patterns do not allow for night shifts (24-hour system, night work only, 2 x 12.).
- modification of the workstation by the occupational physician because of certain chronic pathologies that contraindicate night work.
- no on-call system in the establishment.

The 24-hour system, which is very demanding, has been introduced in certain remote structures that lack transport (e.g. rural areas) and in university hospitals (e.g. emergency services).
81.9% of our doctors felt they were overworked. This result was almost similar among private practitioners in the Ile-de-France region (89.1%) [126], but higher than that of a Canadian study (64%) [127]. In the latter study, doctors worked on average between 50 and 60 hours per week [127].
The workload considered heavy by our sample can probably not be due to the number of hours worked, since the average was only 31.4 ± 5.4 hours per week. It could be due to other factors, such as the aggressiveness of citizens, the injustice felt, and the atmosphere within the team.
On the other hand, numerous surveys have shown that excessive working hours do not necessarily lead to an increase in productivity, but rather tend to reduce the effectiveness and efficiency of individuals [128]. Furthermore, while overwork can be harmful to workers' mental health, the same is true of underwork, which can lead to boredom and a drop in motivation and job satisfaction [129].
In the literature, it was above all the perceived workload that had an influence on the desire to change profession and not the objective workload (number of hours worked per week, number of shifts per month, etc.) [130].
When the pace of work is fast and it is necessary to manage a continuous, tense flow as well as difficult, complex or urgent situations, it is difficult to cope with this situation [110, 131].
Work overload was significantly related to gender ($p<0.05$). This could be explained by the fact that, in addition to their work, women had significant family commitments.
With regard to decision-making, we found that only 2% of GPs in the PHCs did not take their decisions independently, compared with 26.9% of those practising in hospitals. The latter had to seek the advice of a resident, a specialist or a university hospitalist. There was a highly significant relationship between structure and autonomy in decision-making ($p<0.001$).
The majority of GPs (86%) said that they had been attacked since they started practising. This figure was significantly lower for those practising in rural areas ($p<0.01$). In fact, 46.2% of doctors who practised in rural areas had not been attacked, compared with 15.4% who worked in urban areas, which can probably be explained by the respect that rural people always show doctors. The assaults reported were verbal or physical, from patients or their relatives.
Attacks, which occurred mainly at night or during on-call duty, were very unpopular with our

practitioners. In a study of 1,093 British GPs, it was reported that 63% had experienced some form of aggression in the 12 months preceding the survey [132]. The Observatoire de l'insécurité en France also recorded the same rate of verbal aggression (62%) among GPs [110].

Physical aggression was 5% in our population, and 13% in France [110]. A much higher rate was found in a study of 567 general practitioners in the Netherlands, 25% of whom said they had been physically threatened in the year preceding the survey [133]. A French study also showed that problematic relations with patients had a greater impact on professional fatigue than workload [47]. This phenomenon of difficulties in relations between doctors and patients is new, since it rarely existed 40 years ago [134].

More than half of our practitioners (53.1%) felt injustice mainly from the administration (84.1% of cases), followed by their specialist colleagues. A study also reported this situation of injustice by Belgian GPs who complained of being treated in a haughty manner by their specialist colleagues [46].

Almost half of our sample (48.2%) found the working atmosphere to be average.

87.9% of doctors said they could count on support in the event of a problem, especially from their family (83.3%), colleagues (68.6%) or friends (45.9%). The people who provide the most comfort are their families.

78% of our doctors said they were not satisfied with their salary given the high cost of living; this rate was almost identical among Belgian GPs, 75% of whom thought they were poorly remunerated [46].

84% of GPs had attended medical training courses, and almost all of the sample (99%) recognised the need for such training in order to update their knowledge. For the 16% of GPs who had never attended training courses, the reasons given were: distance, inconvenient timetables, unsatisfactory quality of training and, for some, the absence of such training at their practice.

VI.1.3 Characteristics of GPs' private lives

64% of GPs stated that they had no personal or family problems, although they were unable to devote enough time to their family in 52% of cases, or to have time for extra-professional activities in 59% of cases.

In the literature, 84% of self-employed doctors in the Paris region complained of a lack of time for their private lives [126] and 39% of Luxembourg GPs said they did not devote enough time to their loved ones [37].

VI.2 IMPACT OF PROFESSIONAL ACTIVITY ON THE POPULATION STUDIED

60.7% of GPs drank coffee, in quantities ranging from 1 to 8 cups a day, and for periods of up to 40 years.

3.7% were male smokers. This result was lower than the rate found among 306 GPs in the Loire département, which was 14% [3]. In 2008, 18% of French GPs said they were smokers, with an over-representation of men [135].

As these addictive behaviours are taboo in our society, none of the women admitted to smoking, and none of the doctors admitted to taking drugs or alcohol.

16% of those questioned admitted to having taken or still taking psychotropic drugs, mainly to sleep or to combat anxiety. In more than 2/3 of cases (67.6%), this was self-medication. An identical rate of consumption (15.9%) was reported in a French study of general medical interns, but self-medication was higher (81.1%) [79].

Our doctors therefore do not consult their colleagues and treat themselves, even when it

comes to this category of drugs. This phenomenon was also observed in France[98].
In a French study, it was reported that 30.4% of patients took psychotropic drugs, i.e. double the rate observed in our study [3], whereas in a Moroccan study of anaesthetic and intensive care staff, the rate was much lower (5.2%) [136].
We therefore agree with some [125] that doctors most often resort to denial, the use of psychoactive substances and self-medication.
The average number of hours of sleep per night was 6.5. An almost identical result was found among Luxembourg GPs (6.8 hours) [37]. In our study, 52.8% of the women complained most about sleep problems. This could be explained by the fact that women slept less than men (20.1% vs. 12.9% for a number of hours of sleep < 5).
Sick leave was significantly related to gender ($p<0.001$). In fact, 41.4% of female doctors compared with 18.7% of male doctors had taken one or more sick leaves.
Less than a quarter (23.5%) of our population presented no somatic complaints, while the rest of the sample reported one or more at a time. Doctors in Luxembourg reported none in 60.5% of cases [37]. The most frequent complaint observed among our GPs was chronic fatigue (48.8%), as reported in the literature [15]; this rate was lower among anaesthetists in Morocco [136]. The other complaints found among our doctors were, in order of frequency: digestive disorders, musculoskeletal pain, headaches, neurovegetative disorders and precordialgia.
The majority (84.4%) of GPs were afraid of committing a medical error, especially during on-call duty or when they were overwhelmed.
In a survey conducted in Canada, the fear of medical error appears to be a factor that causes distress and burnout among doctors. According to them, committing a medical error exposes them to professional reprimand, punishment by peers, the possibility of disbarment, and even legal action [137]. This fear and distress can have serious consequences. Indeed, several doctors committed suicide in France in 2011 because they were involved in proven or perceived medical errors [110].
More than half of our doctors (56.8%) said they regretted having studied so long and so hard to end up in this situation. Similar results (57.9%) were found among American doctors who said they would not recommend medicine as a career to their children or to other young people, and more than 1/3 would not do medicine again if they had the choice.
In our study, 43.4% of GPs expressed a desire to change profession. A lower rate was observed in Luxembourg (21.2%) [37] and Morocco (39.3%) [136], but a higher rate (58%) in the Loire region [3]. This desire to change profession is considered by some to be a warning sign of burnout [123, 139].
5% of doctors had had suicidal thoughts (3 men and 20 women), none of whom had actually acted on them, compared with 8.3% of GPs on the island of Réunion [135], 13% of those working in the Loire region of France [3] and 10.8% of GPs in Luxembourg [37]. Among Swiss doctors, this rate was higher (1/3 out of a sample of 3,000 primary care doctors) [140]. A lower result (2.1%) was reported by a Moroccan study among staff in anaesthesia-intensive care departments at four university hospitals (doctors, teachers, specialists, residents and nurses constituted the target study population) [136].
This low rate among our respondents and among the Maghrebi population in general could be explained by the fact that this phenomenon is taboo and also by religious considerations (Islam condemns suicide).
This question surprised most of the doctors questioned, who answered with a surprised "never".

Only 26.1% of our GPs (slightly more than 1/4) had heard of OBE or burnout syndrome. This rate was higher among general medical interns in France (89.3%), but lower (15%) in a study of practitioners in French hospitals [141]. The fact that doctors do not identify this syndrome is a major defect in their perception of it, leading to a poor ability to identify their own state of suffering [141].

It should be noted that courses on OB are not included in the curriculum for medical students, whereas they are an integral part of the programme for paramedical students.

VI.3 PREVALENCE OF BO AND ITS THREE DIMENSIONS

Studies	Population	High EE (%)	High PD (%)	Low AP (%)	Severe BO (%)	BO present (%)	No BO/low (%)
Our study (n=463)	MG	37,8	12,3	17,7	3,2	49	16
Sidi Bel Abbes (n=168)[9]	resident doctors	95,2	75	59,1			
Morocco (n=290)[142]	doctors & nurses	48,2	21,3	42,7		69,6	30,3
Morocco (n=191) [143]	doctors in training[3]	63,5	55,6	73	31,8		
Tunisia (n=113)[144]	MG	35	21	40	7,1	33	
Tunisia (n=100) [145]	doctors & nurses	47	36,6	33		56	
Tunisia (n=342)[146]	young doctors[a]	62,9	71,6	56,1		28,7	
Senegal (n=192) [147]	resident doctors	64	45,2	84,9	11,8		
France (n=306)[3]	MG	26	34	19	5		16
France (n=259) [34]	MG	47,9	40	37			
France (n=408)[47]	specialists and generalists	42,3	44,5	37,4			
France (n=511)[148]	MG	23	19,6	10,6	1		25
France (n=4050) [5]	interns in general medicine	16	33,8	38,9	6,5		41,9
France ile de la reunion (n=120)[135]	MG	20	21	18	3,6		
France (n=130)[149]	MG	26,2	22,3	20	6,9	46	54
Studies	**Population**	**High EE (%)**	**High PD (%)**	**Low AP (%)**	**Severe BO (%)**	**BO present (%)**	**No BO/low (%)**
Luxembourg (n=157)[37]	MG	10,8	12,1	33,1	1,9		15,2
12 European countries	MG	43	35,3	32	12		35,1

(n=1393)[123]							
Italy (n=328)[7]	MG	32,4	27,4	13,1			
Portugal (n=150) [150]	MG	25,3	16,2	16,7	2		
Switzerland (n=1755) [6]	MG	19	22	16	3,5		
Denmark (n=216)[151]	MG	14,8	10,2	25,5	3,7		
Yemen (n=563)[152]	doctors	63,2	19,4	33	11,7		
Saudi Arabia (n=144)[153]	MG	53,5	38,9	28,5	2,7		24,3
Dubai (n=102)[154]	MG	42,6	13,7	45			
7 Arab countries (19 studies) (n=4108)[155]	health professionals	20-81	9,2-80	13,3-85,8			
Brazil (n=127)[156]	healthcare professionals	36,2	15,7	7,9			
Brazil (n=297)[157]	doctors	47,5	24,6	28,3	7,4		
USA (n=7288)[158]	doctors	37,9	29,4	12,4		45,8	

a: interns and residents

Table 32 Comparison of the prevalences of OB and its 3 dimensions with other studies studies

In order to compare prevalences, it is important to have a similar treatment of responses; we therefore only selected studies which used the same assessment tool (MBI) with its three dimensions (EE, DP and AP), which targeted populations of doctors or other healthcare professionals but which also included a population of doctors in their sample. According to Maslach and his colleagues, the individual does not have an overall burnout score; each dimension must be interpreted according to its score; a high level of burnout in one dimension is enough to affirm its existence[40]. For others, burnout can be exploited globally as a single syndrome[55].

In this work, we will compare the prevalence of OO found in our sample with that of other studies, but above all we will compare each of the three dimensions separately as recommended by Maslach and his team.

VI.3.1 Burnout

Almost half (49%) of our population were experiencing burnout. Among the authors who calculated this rate in the above studies (table 33), the study carried out in France in the Gers among a population of GPs found a result slightly lower than ours (46%)[149]. A rate of 45.8% was also observed in a population of American doctors made up of GPs and specialists [158], and this author reported that this prevalence was twice as high as in other professions in the USA.

The Moroccan and Tunisian studies reported a higher prevalence of 69.6% [142] and 56% [145] respectively, but both studies involved a sample of doctors and nurses.
Another Tunisian study of young doctors (interns and residents) found a lower rate (28.7%)[146].
In France, the national prevalence of burnout among general practitioners (n=221) was estimated at 51.5% in 2007 (study not mentioned in the table), a rate almost identical to that in our study [159].
Concerning the absence of BO (low EE, low DP and high AP), our study reported a low rate of 16%. The same result was observed among French GPs in the Loire department [3], and a similar result (15.2%) among Luxembourg doctors[37].This prevalence was higher in the other studies that calculated this rate.

VI.3.2 Severe burnout

3.2% of our doctors had a high level of burnout (all three components simultaneously high EE, high DP and low AP). For the studies that calculated this rate, it was lower in French doctors (general practitioners)[148], Luxembourg doctors[37], Portuguese doctors[150] and Saudi doctors[153], ranging from 1% to 2.7%.
Prevalences almost identical to our result were observed among doctors at in Switzerland [6], France (Ile de la Réunion) [135] and Denmark [151].
The highest prevalence (31.8%) was observed in a population of Moroccan doctors in training (interns and residents)[143].

V I.3.3 Emotional exhaustion

In our study, the prevalence of EE was 37.8%. This rate was low compared with the study carried out in the west of the country, which was 95% [9]. However, this was a population of resident doctors who, in addition to their work, had to study and prepare for examinations, which probably represents an additional constraint and stress. We also noted that, even in the Tunisian[146], Moroccan[143] and Senegalese[147] studies, this rate exceeded 60% in each case, as these were residents.
In a systematic review of 19 studies carried out in 7 Arab countries (Maghreb countries not included)[155], where the prevalence of EE varied from 20 to 81% depending on the study, the highest rate (81%) was found in an Egyptian study which also involved this category of doctor. However, in a French sample of 4050 general medical interns, we observed a low rate of EE (16%)[5].
Comparing the prevalence of emotional exhaustion in our sample with that found in studies of GPs, this rate was close to that found in Tunisia (35%)[144], but higher than in other European studies [3, 6, 7, 37, 135, 148151]. The American study, which looked at a population of GPs and specialists, reported the same rate (37.9%)[158].
However, our doctors were less exhausted than doctors practising in Dubai[154], Yemen[152], Saudi Arabia[153] and Brazil[157], as well as in the study of GPs from 12 European countries[123].

V I.3.4 Depersonalisation

The prevalence rate of PD among our GPs was among the lowest compared with these different studies. Indeed, the rate of 12.3% was close to the study carried out among Danish GPs (10.2%)[151] and Luxembourg GPs (12.1%)[37].We also observed that the highest rates were observed among resident doctors. The lowest rate (9.2%) reported in the systematic review was observed in a sample of Palestinian nurses[155].
We may think that this low prevalence rate observed in our population could be due to the

human and warm-hearted side of the individual generally known in our society, to our doctor's significant involvement in the emotional relationship with patients, despite all the difficulties of the medical profession, the injustices felt and the aggression of certain patients or some of their relatives.

V I.3.5 Personal achievement

The 17.7% prevalence rate of PA was close to that observed among GPs on Reunion Island (18%)[135].our doctors were more accomplished than their North African, Arab (Gulf countries) or African (Senegal) colleagues. The Brazilian study[156] reported the lowest prevalence rate (7.9%) and therefore the best personal achievement; however, it should be noted that this was a population which included all healthcare professionals.

Our doctors were less accomplished compared with their colleagues in Europe (France, Italy, Switzerland and Portugal)[6, 7, 148, 150] and the United States[158]; lack of resources and inadequate training could perhaps explain this feeling of inefficiency and devaluation. However, there are some European studies and a Brazilian study [157] in which the PA rate among their doctors was lower than in our sample.

At the end of this comparison, we were able to observe that the results concerning the prevalence of this syndrome vary in the literature from one country to another and even within the same country. Most authors believe that this variability in results could be explained by methodological, socio-economic and professional differences in the samples studied (culture, lifestyle, working conditions, etc.).

V I.4 FACTORS ASSOCIATED WITH BURNOUT

V I.4.1 Factors associated with high emotional exhaustion

V I.4.1.1 High emotional exhaustion and characteristics of the population studied

V I.4.1.1.1 High EE and socio-demographic characteristics

In the literature, the data on the influence of gender on this dimension are discordant: while some studies incriminate the female sex as being at greater risk [3, 160], others have found it to be lower in women [47, 161, 162], while a third group found no link [7, 31, 150, 163].

In our study, we found no significant link between high EE and gender.

The greater vulnerability of women reported by some may be related to their greater involvement in the emotional relationship with their patients and to the difficulty of reconciling their professional and family lives [164]. Other authors attribute this to the psychobiological characteristics of women, who have more emotional and empathetic attitudes, unlike men, who tend to have more instrumental attitudes [165].

The authors who found an association between the male sex and burnout [162] attributed this to the greater workload given to men.

Age had no influence on this dimension in our population or in most others [3, 7, 47, 163].

As in some studies [7, 15, 161], marital status had no influence on this dimension in our study. However, some authors believe that being married is a protective factor against burnout; spousal support could play a role in preventing difficulties and problems arising in everyday life as well as at work [166].

The number of children was not related to EE. This result has also been observed in the literature [3, 15, 31].

Moreira et al. found an association between burnout and being a young woman, aged between 26 and 35, married, without children and working for more than five years [167].

Our chronically ill doctors were significantly emotionally exhausted. This result was also observed in Kuwait among a population of doctors practising in basic care centres [168].

Since emotional exhaustion is defined as severe fatigue felt in an unusual way and which is not, or is only slightly, improved by rest [15], a doctor with a pathology will be much more exhausted, and to a greater extent.

V I.4.1.1.2 High EE and professional activity characteristics

Among our GPs, working in a hospital was significantly associated with EE. This result was also observed in an Iranian study [161], while according to an Italian study [7], the hospital is a less stressful environment and the doctor is in a better protected environment.

We can explain our result by the fact that our doctors, who treat mainly in-patients in hospitals, would be less autonomous and would feel unfairly treated by their specialist or university hospital colleagues.

Doctors who worked in rural areas were less emotionally exhausted, and this was highly significant, which is in line with the results of a study carried out on general medical interns in France [5]. On the other hand, the results of another study showed that practising medicine in a rural environment tended (although not significantly) to generate high EE, and to foster conflict and strained relations with patients [47]. Among GPs in the Loire and Gers regions of France, no link was observed [3, 149].

The number of years in practice had no influence on emotional exhaustion, as observed elsewhere [3].

We found that doctors who arrived late for work were significantly more exhausted than others. We believe that lateness could have negative consequences; the doctor would have to carry out his work in a reduced time, deal with the anger of patients and suffer the reproaches of the administration, leading to exhaustion.

Doctors working less than 30 hours a week had an EE rate of 35.4%, rising to 44.9% when the number of hours exceeded 39, but this was not significant. A French study of 978 doctors working in intensive care units also reported that emotional exhaustion was not related to the number of hours worked [169]. Galam's study of a sample of 4050 general medical interns in France reported that those who worked an average of 47.2 hours per week did not suffer from OBE, whereas those who worked more (48.7 hours per week) had one of the three pathological OBE scores with a highly significant association [5]. Swiss doctors who worked more than 50 hours a week were exposed to high burnout [170].

A Taiwanese study reported that working overtime up to 80 hours/month for 6 months increased the risk of dying from *Karoshi* (Japanese term for death from overwork). Seven doctors died in Taiwan from *Karoshi between 2008 and 2012.* Seven doctors died in Taiwan from *karoshi* during the period from 2008 to 2012[171].the link, which was not significant in our population, could be explained by the fact that the number of hours per week did not exceed 45.

Work overload, which was significantly associated with this dimension in our study, is in line with results found elsewhere [3, 26, 148, 172].

Care workers who felt that there was an incompatibility between their workload and their salaries had a higher risk of burnout than those who were satisfied with their salaries [173].

The causal relationship between burnout and excessive workload is reciprocal. Indeed, it could be that carers suffering from burnout increase their workload to compensate for the feeling of failure [174].

Not being autonomous in decision-making led to high EE, and burnout in general [26], since depriving doctors of autonomy during their practice is a major determinant of job dissatisfaction [175]. This result was also observed in our research.

Our doctors reported mainly verbal aggression from patients and their parents, but also physical aggression. Being confronted with patients' aggressiveness and aggression seems to be a major cause of emotional exhaustion in our study, as well as in the study carried out at Constantine University Hospital on a sample of 442 people (190 doctors and 295 paramedics) [176].

51.2% of GPs who were emotionally exhausted felt injustice compared with 22.6% in the opposite case; injustice therefore generates a high EE.

A poor working atmosphere and conflicts within the team were a major source of burnout. This result has also been reported among doctors working in intensive care units in France [169].

The opportunity to update their knowledge and follow ongoing medical training was associated with a lower rate of burnout among Danish GPs [2], but this link was not observed in our population.

VI.4.1.3 High EE and privacy characteristics

Our results showed significantly that insufficient time devoted to the family and the existence of personal or family problems were associated with a high score. This was also observed in a population of general practitioners in Provence-Alpes-Côte d'Azur [148] and in Luxembourg [37].

A study published in the Netherlands on work-life interference showed that work had an influence on family life, and vice versa. The existence of a conflict between these two components will therefore have a major influence on the onset of burnout [177], and is also one of the major causes of this syndrome [124, 178].

VI.4.1.2 High EE and impact of professional activity on the population studied

With regard to addictive behaviours, in our study as in others [3, 121], the use of psychotropic drugs was linked to emotional exhaustion. This use may be induced by the exhaustion of the doctor, who seeks refuge in these substances, which will help him to detach himself temporarily from his worries. However, the use of these substances can alter the quality of medical practice and the doctor's personal and professional perceptions, leading to BO [8].

Our emotionally exhausted GPs had sleep disorders in 49.1% of cases. A higher rate (74.1%) was observed in general medical interns[79].

This syndrome is generally linked to absenteeism [26], a result that we did not observe in our study.

In our work, doctors who reported somatic complaints were emotionally exhausted in 44.9% of cases compared with 14.7% of cases for those who did not complain. In Tunisia, this link was also observed in two studies [145, 179].

41.2% of doctors with a high EE were afraid of making medical errors. An even higher rate (83%) was reported among general practitioners working in health centres in Finland [180]. In a study in Morocco of medical and paramedical staff in anaesthesia-intensive care departments, fear of medical error was significantly linked to burnout in general [142].This link was also observed among Taiwanese doctors [171].

Exhausted doctors were no longer satisfied with their work and wanted to change profession [3, 37, 121, 144, 153].This finding was also significant in our sample. In a study of 11530 healthcare professionals in Spain and Latin America, there was a very strong association between this component and the desire to leave one's profession [181]. It is quite normal for emotional exhaustion to appear or worsen when doctors continue to work in a profession they no longer enjoy [37].

Exhausted doctors risk leaving the profession, thereby reducing access to care[182].
For suicidal ideation, contrary to the literature [3, 135], we did not observe any association in our study.

V **I.4.2 Factors associated with high depersonalisation**

V I.4.2.1 High PD and characteristics of the population studied

V I.4.2.1.1 High PD and socio-demographic characteristics

In some studies, women depersonalised their patients less than men [7, 37, 47, 148, 150, 161], while in others, there was no influence of gender [3]. A study carried out in Egypt among doctors practising in a university hospital, on the other hand, found that it was women who had a higher PD [183].

Age and marital status were not associated with PD [7].

In our study, only the number of children was associated with a high level of depersonalisation. Those with two or fewer children had a significantly higher PD than those with more (14% vs. 8.9%). In Senegal, in a population of residents, there was a highly significant link between this dimension and not having any children [147].

V I.4.2.1.2 High PD and professional activity characteristics

Working in a hospital had an influence on this dimension in our study as well as in the one carried out in Iran [161], unlike the study carried out among French doctors in the Loire department, which found no association with place of work [3]. In Egypt, a study reported that doctors who worked in hospitals were 10 times more likely to develop burnout than other doctors [183]. We believe that it is in hospitals that GPs are most confronted with pain and death, and therefore develop impersonal and cynical attitudes towards hospital patients in order to cope with the exhaustion of their internal resources. Professionals who previously "over-identified" with the suffering of these patients begin to deny their original motivation and detach themselves from the ethical significance of the act of care [184]. According to some, this attitude is a way of adapting to the collapse of motivation and energy [34].

Our results are in line with those of certain studies which found no link between this dimension and the number of years of exercise [7].

Doctors suffering from depersonalisation no longer feel concerned by their work [34], which could explain the delay in work reported by our GPs who had a high PD.

GPs who felt that their workload was heavy significantly depersonalised their patients more. A national survey of 2536 Canadian doctors also reported this link [185].

In our study, doctors who had been attacked depersonalised their patients to a much greater extent than those who had not (13.8% vs. 3.1%), as did those who felt injustice in the workplace. A study of 809 Taiwanese doctors reported that dissatisfaction with the doctor-patient relationship was a highly significant source of depersonalisation [171]. The poor working environment was also a source of dehumanisation and cynicism. According to some[186], organisation, work atmosphere and lack of support are very important determinants of OB and are most often found in surveys.

V I.4.2.1.3 High PD and privacy characteristics

GPs who did not devote enough time to their families, or who had personal or family problems, had a high PD rate.

V I.4.2.2 High PD and impact of professional activity on the population studied

There was an association with the use of psychotropic drugs, as in the study of resident doctors in Sidi Bel-Abbes [9] and the study of general practitioners in Saudi Arabia [153].

The link between sleep disorders and high burnout in general has often been reported using subjective or objective assessment methods. In a study of 240 Spanish doctors [187], this relationship was objectified by the *Pittsburgh score,* translated and validated in Spanish. The Pittsburgh Sleep Quality Index (PSQI) is an instrument used to screen for sleep disorders; it is

one of the few assessment instruments to combine both the quantitative and qualitative components of sleep. The original version is in English [188], and the questionnaire has been validated and translated into French [189].
In our study, where sleep disorders were assessed subjectively, this link was also observed.
We found that the complaints reported by our doctors were very positively associated with depersonalisation.
The study of doctors practising in 12 European countries reported a significant link between this dimension and work stoppages [123], a result which we did not observe in our work.
13.3% of our doctors who depersonalised their patients were afraid of committing a medical error. In a national survey of 7509 surgeons in the USA, those with severe depersonalisation had a very high probability of committing a serious medical error [190].
Our results showed that doctors who did not want to go back to medical school were more likely to depersonalise their patients.
A high level of depersonalisation was associated with the desire for reconversion in our study as well as in others. [3, 123, 191].
High PD was associated with suicidal ideation in our doctors and those on the island of Réunion [135]. This association was not observed among doctors in the Loire region [3].
In our study, depression was not assessed using specific scales, but among the perceived consequences, feelings of low self-esteem and suicidal ideation were correlated with burnout. Indeed, confusion between burnout syndrome and depression is common [164]. Some authors have even assumed that burnout is a form of depression [165]. In this way, burnout syndrome can be a precursor to full-blown major depression and can even lead to suicide.
However, as our doctors did not specify the period in their lives when these suicidal thoughts occurred, we cannot say whether these thoughts are the consequence of this depersonalisation.

V I.4.3 Factors associated with low personal fulfilment

V I.4.3.1 Low PA and characteristics of the population studied

V I.4.3.1.1 Low PA and socio-demographic characteristics

In our GPs, the personal achievement score was not related to sex, which has also been described by other authors [47]. In Portuguese and Egyptian studies, male doctors had lower PA scores [150, 183].
At the start of their careers, our doctors under the age of 35 felt that they were not effective, that they were not doing a good job, which led to a low PA rate. An association between age and this dimension has also been observed among Taiwanese doctors [171]. A study carried out in a hospital in Kuwait on doctor satisfaction reported that the youngest and least experienced doctors had the lowest satisfaction scores [192]. Another study of 192 Senegalese residents found a lower rate of personal fulfilment in those under 30 [147]. In our study, from the age of 45 onwards, we observed a clear improvement in this rate of personal fulfilment; the older residents had revised their aspirations and acquired skills and effective means of coping.
Being single or married had no influence on this dimension in our study. In Kuwait, a study reported that not being married led to low PA among doctors [168]. In contrast, in France, there was an association between living with a partner and low self-fulfilment among urban GPs. The authors of this survey were surprised by this result, which contradicts the hypothesis of the moderating effect of social support in the appearance of this phenomenon. They explained this observation by the fact that long working days and weeks could lead to a reduced opportunity for support from spouses [148].

The number of children had an influence on this dimension. We found that looking after two or fewer children led to lower levels of personal fulfilment. According to some, having dependent children seems to be a protective factor against burnout because they can be a resource. They may also represent an additional motivation to work [37]. We believe that in our sample, fulfilment would appear for doctors with more than two children.

V I.4.3.1.2 Low PA and professional activity characteristics

In this study, there was a significant association between the number of years in practice and the decline in PA. The rate was 23% in GPs who had practised for five years or less, which is consistent with the idea that there is a loss of idealism among doctors during the first years of practice, which could lead to burnout [193]. We may think that a doctor's lack of experience could initially encourage a decline in personal fulfilment. However, this length of professional practice remains controversial. While several authors have found that burnout is negatively correlated with professional experience [194], others have stated that burnout is more prevalent in those with more professional experience. Montero specified that burnout was significantly more frequent in staff who had been working for more than sixteen years [195].

The results showed that doctors who were attacked had a lower PA. We believe that aggression is a source of demotivation.

GPs who rated their working environment as average had a significantly lower rate of personal achievement than those who rated it as good or bad. This result may surprise us insofar as it is usually poor working conditions that lead to demotivation.

Among doctors who did not attend medical training, 26.3% had a low PA compared with 16% for those who had attended training courses, with a significant link. Updating their knowledge and improving their skills could help practitioners avoid this feeling of inefficiency and self-deprecation.

By updating their knowledge, doctors can improve their relationship with patients, provide them with better care and promote their knowledge to them. This training will also help them to break their isolation and can therefore represent a real resource for them [37]. It would be difficult for low-level PA doctors to invest in the smooth running of their work.

V I.4.3.1.3 Low AP and privacy characteristics

Not having enough time for oneself (extra-professional activities: leisure or other) or for one's family were significantly associated with low PA. These results are in line with those of doctors in Luxembourg, Senegalese resident doctors and general medical interns in the Ile de France region [37, 121, 147]. When doctors are in burnout, they tend to work too hard ("presenteeism") and do not spend much time with those close to them whose role is to value their profession. It is this appreciation that will contribute to the existence of a high sense of accomplishment.

V I.4.3.2 Low PA and impact of professional activity on the population studied

Addictive behaviour, fear of medical error and suicidal thoughts were not linked to this dimension.

Doctors who complained of sleep problems had a lower PA.

In our study, GPs who did not want to go back to medical school or who felt the need to retrain were very significantly low in personal fulfilment. In the literature, the desire to retrain was also associated with a low level of personal fulfilment [3, 37, 123].

V I.5 MULTIVARIATE ANALYSIS

The logistic regression model used explained 83.4% of the variance in the occurrence of emotional exhaustion and 83.4% of the variance in personal fulfilment, which is considered

very satisfactory. On the other hand, with regard to feelings of depersonalisation, the model explained only 14.4% of the variance.
Our multivariate analysis showed that GPs with a heavy workload, somatic complaints, fear of making a medical error, use of psychotropic drugs, who worked in urban areas and those who felt a sense of injustice were more likely to have a high EE. On the other hand, those who worked in a hospital, with a good team and who did not want to go back to medical school were less likely to experience EE.
Among the factors predictive of emotional exhaustion in Luxembourg GPs and in a population composed of Tunisian doctors and nurses, there was excessive workload with an OR= 4.9 and an OR=3.80 respectively[37, 145] , which is in line with the result of our study (OR=4.50). In a study of 1784 Swiss GPs, the predictors identified as being associated with a high degree of burnout were gender (men), practice in rural areas, stress related to heavy workload, economic constraints, uncertainty surrounding medical care and relations with non-medical staff[6].Some of these factors were not addressed in our questionnaire. There was no link between gender and this dimension in our study, whereas for work area, it was rather practice in an urban area that was associated with this dimension in our GPs.
GPs who felt the need to retrain and who arrived late for work were more likely to develop a high level of depersonalisation. On the other hand, this feeling was less likely among those who devoted time to their family or who worked in a team under good conditions. Belkhouja et al. found in their study that female gender was a predictive factor in the occurrence of high burnout [196], whereas in the French study conducted in 2006, the multivariate analysis showed that female gender was protective against depersonalisation [159]. In our work, there was no link with gender.
In a Tunisian study of doctors and nurses[145], lack of free time (OR=3.54) was one of the factors predicting a high level of depersonalisation.
For low PA, it was found among GPs who had fewer than two children and those who felt the need to retrain (OR =2.60). The desire to change careers was also observed among GPs in Luxembourg (OR =3.16) [37].
In the European study (12 countries) [123], the factors that were found to be independently associated with depersonalisation and personal fulfilment were the need to retrain, a result that we observed in our GPs.
The study carried out in Morocco on doctors and nurses in the anaesthesia and intensive care departments of 4 university hospitals reported that the causes of burnout in general were professional status (OR 2.77 for resident doctors and 2.63 for nurses), lack of organisation within the department (OR 1.88), fear of medical error (OR 2.09) and unsatisfactory pay/effort ratio (OR 1.93)[142].
In Tunisia, the factors that were independently associated with the risk of developing burnout in young doctors were the absence of leisure activities (OR=2.1) [146].

CONCLUSION

This study enabled us to assess the prevalence of burnout among general practitioners practising in the health and hospital facilities of the Wilaya of Sétif, which was 49%. Severe burnout, where all three dimensions were affected, was 3.2%. Emotional exhaustion affected 37.8%, depersonalisation (which some authors prefer to call dehumanisation) 12.3%, and personal fulfilment 17.7%. With these rates, our doctors are more emotionally exhausted than published studies, depersonalise their patients less and are more accomplished, especially compared with their North African and Arab (Gulf countries) colleagues.

Several factors were linked to the three dimensions of OB in the univariate analysis.

At the end of the multivariate analysis, and in order to adjust the effect of the variables in relation to each other and to take account of any confounding effects, the factors that were independently associated with the three dimensions of burnout in doctors :

- heavy workload, somatic complaints, fear of making a medical error, use of psychotropic drugs, working in an urban area, and a sense of injustice for emotional exhaustion.
- the need to retrain and arriving late for work were predictive of a high level of depersonalisation.
- the least personally accomplished GPs felt the need to retrain. Curiously, we also found this feeling among those caring for fewer than two children.

Workload, whether subjective or objectified in certain studies by the number of patients examined, for example, appears to be the major risk factor for emotional exhaustion (OR 4.50 with $p = 0.0001$).

The consequences of burnout seemed to be somatic complaints, fear of committing a medical error, and the use of psychotropic drugs in the EE dimension. The desire to change profession linked with the DP and AP dimensions may also be one of the consequences of burnout.

Like most authors, we believe that a cross-sectional study cannot establish a causal link, but can nevertheless give an indication of the factors linked to OB.

This syndrome does not seem to be a public health concern in Algeria, but solutions to this scourge should be sought, as its consequences would be damaging for both doctors and patients in the short and long term. Despite the existence of occupational medicine departments in various health establishments across the country, our practitioners almost never consult them, which is why it is so difficult to identify doctors in difficulty at the onset of symptoms and to treat them. In some countries, burnout is recognised as an occupational disease, while in others doctors are struggling to get it recognised.

The creation of discussion groups in care facilities for sharing experiences would be interesting and could be a way of supporting GPs' professional well-being.

Our study therefore provided an overview of burnout syndrome in the Wilaya of Sétif. It would be desirable for similar surveys to be generalised throughout the country and extended to other health professionals. Finally, we hope that this work can serve as a basis for raising awareness of this reality in the field among doctors, supervisory authorities and higher authorities, so that an action plan can be drawn up to deal effectively with this health phenomenon.

RECOMMENDATIONS AND OUTLOOK

At the end of our study, and in order to prevent early burnout, the extreme manifestation of which is burnout syndrome, we have attempted to draw up the following recommendations:

- Inclusion of modules on the subject of OB in the university curriculum for medical students.
- Training medical students and raising their awareness of this health phenomenon.
- Compulsory continuing medical education to update medical knowledge.
- The need to work in a group during the first years of a doctor's posting (responsibility exercised in isolation can contribute to the development of the OB).
- The need to develop initiatives to inform the general public and the media about the importance and complexity of the GP's role. Without forgetting to highlight the constraints and limitations of the practitioner's job in the field.
- Effective implementation of ministerial instruction no. 18 of 27 October 2002 relating to the protection of the health of healthcare workers [197] (appendix 6), which is subject to :
- the human and material resources required for its application.
- analysis of work activities and working conditions.
- medico-environmental monitoring in healthcare environments.
- the involvement of occupational health departments, which must :
- *S* systematically visit all care staff,
- *S* focus their activities more on risk assessment and prevention.
- buy-in from managers, staff and employee representatives
- Recognition of the arduous nature of the medical profession.

BIBLIOGRAPHICAL REFERENCES

1. WINCKLER M, . La maladie de Sachs: Paris, P.O.L; 1998.
2. Brandt A, Sokolowski I, Olesen F, Vedsted P. Continuing medical education and burnout among Danish GPs. British Journal of General Practice. 2008;58:15-9.
3. Cathébras P, Begon A, Laporte S, Bois C, Truchot D. Burnout among general practitioners. La Presse Médicale. 2004;33(22):1569-74.
4. Dyrbye LN, Varkey P, Boone SL, Satele DV, Sloan JA, Shanafelt TD. Physician Satisfaction and Burnout at Different Career Stages. Mayo Clinic Proceedings. 2013;88(12): 1358-67.
5. Galam E, Komly V, Le Tourneur A, Jund J. Burnout among French GPs in training: a cross-sectional study. The British journal of general practice : the journal of the Royal College of General Practitioners. 2013;63(608):e217-24. Epub 2013/04/09.
6. Goehring C, Bouvier Gallacchi M, Kunzi B, Bovier P. Psychosocial and professional characteristics of burnout in Swiss primary care practitioners: a cross-sectional survey. Swiss medical weekly. 2005;135(7-8):101-8. Epub 2005/04/16.
7. Grassi L, Magnani K. Psychiatric morbidity and burnout in the medical profession: an Italian study of general practitioners and hospital physicians. Psychotherapy and psychosomatics. 2000;69(6):329-34. Epub 2000/11/09.
8. Jonckheer P, Stordeur S, Lebeer G, Roland M, De Schampheleire J, De Troyer M, et al. Burnout among general practitioners: prevention and management. 2011.
9. Kandouci C, Belhadj Z, Bouaza H, Kandouci A. Evaluation of physicians' suffering through analysis of the concept of burnout. JMT SAMT. 2010;16:67-71.
10. Benatia Y. Burnout among emergency nurses. 2008.
11. Benatia Y. The impact of socioprofessional factors on the emergence of burnout in emergency nurses. 2015.
12. Boudarene M. Souffrance au travail et Burn out chez des agents de Police en exercice. A preliminary study. The International Journal of Victimology. 2004.
13. Boulkroune Nora. le syndrome de burnout chez les enseignants du supérieur 2008.
14. Benferhat A. Burn-out syndrome among doctors in disaster situations: the case of the SAMU of Algiers, Blida and Médéa. 2013.
15. Canoui P, Mauranges A. Le burn out à l'hòpital: le syndrome d'épuisement professionnel: Elsevier Health Sciences; 2008.
16. Zawieja P, Guarnieri F. Professional exhaustion: main conceptual, clinical and psychometric approaches. In: edited by Philippe Zawieja and Franck G, editor. Épuisement professionnel : Approches innovantes et pluridisciplinaires: Armand Colin; 2013. p. 11-34 - Chapter 1.
17. Dejours C, Gernet I. Psychopathologie du travail: Elsevier Masson Paris; 2012.
18. Franceschi-Chaix C, Clément J, Therme J. Le syndrome de burn out. Etude clinique et implication en psychopathologie du travail. recherche en soins infirmiers. 1993;32:5-60.
19. Ballester S, Macovei D, Puel C, Soulat J M. Causes & Consequences of burnout professional experience & prevalence of burnout using the Maslach Burnout Inventory: Preliminary approach.
20. Bährer-Kohler S. Burnout for experts: Prevention in the context of living and working: Springer Science & Business Media; 2012.
21. Bradley HB. Community-based Treatment for Young Adult Offenders. Crime & Delinquency. 1969;15(3):359-70.
22. Schaufeli WB, Buunk BP. Professional burnout. Handbook of work and health psychology1996. p. 311-46.
23. Hoffman A. The BURN OUT: When the doors to the void open... Santé conjuguée. 2005(32):37.
24. Freudenberger HJ. Staff Burn-Out. Journal of Social Issues. 1974;30(1):159-65.
25. Boudoukha A-H. Burn-out et traumatismes psychologiques: Dunod; 2009.

26. Maslach C, Schaufeli WB, Leiter MP. Job burnout. Annual review of psychology. 2001;52(1):397-422. Epub 2001/01/10.
27. Freudenberger HJ, Richelson G. Burn-Out: How to Beat the High Cost of Success Books B, editor. New York 1980.
28. Maslach C, Jackson SE. The measurement of experienced burnout. Journal of Organizational Behavior. 1981;2(2):99-113.
29. Cordes CL, Dougherty TW. A Review and an Integration of Research on Job Burnout. Academy of Management Review. 1993;18(4):621-56.
30. Wiertz R. Psychiatres et burnout: étude de la prevalence du syndrome d'épuisement professionnel auprès des psychiatres hospitaliers du Nord Pas De Calais: Thèse de Doctorat en Médecine, Université du droit et de la santé Lille 2, 2012. 224p; 2012.
31. Ernst M. Burnout syndrome among general medical interns at the Strasbourg Faculty of Medicine: prevalence and analysis of 2009 interviews.
32. Pezet-Langevin V. Burnout: mieux connaître l'épuisement professionnel. Hygiène et sécurité du work. 2014;237:6-9.
33. Schaufeli W, Enzmann D. The burnout companion to study and research: a critical analysis: London: Taylor and Francis; 1998.
34. Truchot D. Le burn-out des médecins généralistes : influence de finiquité perçue et de l'orientation communautaire. Annales Médico-psychologiques, revue psychiatrique. 2009;167(6):422-8.
35. Collange J, Tavani JL, Soula MC. Regards croisés sur le burn-out: aspects médicaux et psychologiques. Archives des Maladies Professionnelles et de l'Environnement. 2013;74(1):35- 43.
36. Grebot É. Stress et burnout au travail: identifier, prévenir, guérir: Editions Eyrolles; 2011.
37. Mangen M-H. Study of Burn out among general practitioners in Luxembourg 2007.
38. Josse E. Burn-in and burn-out. 2008. p. 1-12.
39. Perlman B, Hartman EA. Burnout: Summary and future research. Human relations. 1982;35(4):283-305.
40. Maslach C, Jackson S, Leiter MP. Burnout inventory manual. Palo Alto: California; 1996.
41. Neveu JP. EPUISEMENT PROFESSIONNEL : RECHERCHE EXPLORATOIRE EN MILIEU HOSPITALIER. Le Travail Humain. 1996;59(2):173-86.
42. Maslach C, Leiter MP. The truth about burnout: How organizations cause stress and what to do about it. 1997.
43. Direction Générale du Travail. Paris FRA, Institut National de Recherche et de Sécurité. Paris FRA, National Agency for the Improvement of Working Conditions. Lyon FRA. Le syndrome d'épuisement professionnel ou burnout : Mieux comprendre pour mieux agir. Paris: Ministère du Travail de l'Emploi de la Formation professionnelle et du Dialogue social; 2015. 34p. p.
44. Le Tourneur A, Komly V. Burn out of interns in general medicine: state of play and perspectives in metropolitan France [Thèse d'exercice]. Université Joseph Fourier Grenoble 1. 2011.
45. Maslach C. A multidimensional theory of burnout. Theories of organizational stress. 1998;68.
46. Dagrada H, Verbanck P, Kornreich C. Le burn-out du médecin généraliste: Hypothèses étiologiques. Revue medicale de Bruxelles. 2011;32(4):407-12.
47. Truchot D. Burnout among private practitioners in Champagne Ardenne. Research report for URML Champagne-Ardenne. 2002.
48. Dion G, Tessier R. Validation de la traduction de l'Inventaire d'épuisement professionnel de Maslach et Jackson. Canadian Journal of Behavioural Science/Revue canadienne des sciences du comportement. 1994;26(2):210-27.
49. Demerouti E, Bakker AB. The Oldenburg Burnout Inventory: A good alternative to measure burnout and engagement. Handbook of stress and burnout in health care Hauppauge, NY: Nova Science. 2008.
50. Kristensen TS, Borritz M, Villadsen E, Christensen KB. The Copenhagen Burnout Inventory: A

new tool for the assessment of burnout. Work & Stress. 2005;19(3):192-207.
51. Algava E, Chouanière D, Cohidon C, Dubré J-Y, Kittel F, Leclerc A, et al, editors. Stress au travail et santé : situation chez les indépendants: Éditions de l'INSERM; 2011.
52. Maslach C. Burnout, Psychology of A2 - Wright, James D. International Encyclopedia of the Social & Behavioral Sciences (Second Edition). Oxford: Elsevier; 2015. p. 929-32.
53. Schaufeli WB, Bakker AB, Hoogduin K, Schaap C, Kladler A. on the clinical validity of the maslach burnout inventory and the burnout measure. Psychology & health. 2001;16(5):565-82. Epub 2001/09/01.
54. Maslach C, Leiter MP, Schaufeli W. Measuring burnout. 2008.
55. Ahola K, Honkonen T, Isometsä E, Kalimo R, Nykyri E, Aromaa A, et al. The relationship between job-related burnout and depressive disorders-results from the Finnish Health 2000 Study. Journal of Affective Disorders. 2005;88:55-62.
56. Schaufeli WB, Maslach C, Marek T. Historical and conceptual development of burnout. Professional burnout: Recent developments in theory and research. 1993:1-16.
57. Bibeau G. Le burn-out: 10 ans après. Santé mentale au Québec. 1985;10(2):30-43.
58. Larouche LM. Clinical manifestations of burn out among physicians. Santé mentale au Québec. 1985;10(2): 145-50.
59. Leiter MP, Maslach C. Six areas of worklife: a model of the organizational context of burnout. Journal of health and human services administration. 1999;21(4):472-89. Epub 2000/01/06.
60. PEZET-LANGEVIN V, ROLLAND J-P. Caractéristiques des situations de travail, burmout, et attitude de retrait. European review of applied psychology. 1999;49(3):239-48.
61. Gil-Monte PR, Pilaf V. A model of burnout process development: An alternative from appraisal models of stress. COMPORTAMENTO ORGANIZACIONAL E GESTAO. 1998;4(1):165-79.
62. Leiter MP, Maslach C. Burnout and health. Handbook of health psychology. 2000:415-26.
63. Bakker AB, Demerouti E, Verbeke W. Using the job demands-resources model to predict burnout and performance. Human Resource Management. 2004;43(1):83-104.
64. Demerouti E, Bakker AB, Nachreiner F, Schaufeli WB. The job demands-resources model of burnout. The Journal of applied psychology. 2001;86(3):499-512. Epub 2001/06/23.
65. Barbier D. Le syndrome d'épuisement professionnel du soignant. La Presse Médicale. 2004;33(6):394-9.
66. Colombat P, Altmeyer A, Barruel F, Bauchetet C, Blanchard P, Copel L, et al. Syndrome d'épuisement professionnel des soignants. Oncologie. 2011;13(12):845-63.
67. Rolland J-P. L'évaluation de la personnalité: Le modèle en cinq facteurs: Primento; 2013.
68. Mayou R. Burnout. British Medical Journal (Clinical research ed). 1987;295(6593):284-5.
69. Barbaranelli C, Caprara GV, Maslach C. Individuation and the Five Factor Model of personality traits. European Journal of Psychological Assessment. 1997;13(2):75.
70. Goldberg LR. An Alternative Description of Personality: The Big-Five Factor Structure. Journal of Personality. 1990;59(6):1216-29.
71. Costa Jr PT, McCrae RR. Personality in Adulthood: A Six-Year Longitudinal Study of Self-Reports and Spouse Ratings on the NEO Personality Inventory. Journal of personality and social psychology. 1988;54(5):853-63.
72. Swider BW, Zimmerman RD. Born to burnout: A meta-analytic path model of personality, job burnout, and work outcomes. Journal of Vocational Behavior. 2010;76(3):487-506.
73. Costa PT, McCrae RR. Normal personality assessment in clinical practice: The NEO Personality Inventory. Psychological assessment. 1992;4(1):5.
74. Alarcon G, Eschleman KJ, Bowling NA. Relationships between personality variables and burnout: A meta-analysis. Work & Stress. 2009;23(3):244-63.
75. Louw GJ. Burnout, vigour, big five personality traits and social support in a sample of police officers. SA Journal of Industrial Psychology. 2014;40(1):1-13.
76. Maslach C. What have we learned about burnout and health? Psychology & health.

2001;16(5):607-11. Epub 2001/09/01.
77. Houkes I, Janssen PP, de Jonge J, Bakker AB. Personality, Work Characteristics, and Employee Well-Being: A Longitudinal Analysis of Additive and Moderating Effects. Journal of occupational health psychology. 2003;8(1):20-38.
78. ROSSE JG. Conceptualizing the Role of Self-Esteem in the Burnout Process. Group & Organization Studies. 1991;16(4):42f3-451.
79. Thévenet M. Analyse du burn out chez les internes de médecine générale sur la base d'une étude comparative entre l'Ile-de-France et le Languedoc-Roussillon 2011.
80. Bandura A. Self-efficacy in Changing Societies. 1995.
81. Marceau A. Examen des liens entre la violence psychologique au travail et l'épuisement professionnel en milieu hospitalier. 2006.
82. Dejours C, Abdoucheli E, . Theoretical itinerary in occupational psychopathology. Prévenir. 1990; 20:127-49.
83. Cooper CL, Dewe P. Stress: A brief history: John Wiley & Sons; 2008.
84. Hobfoll SE. Conservation of Resources. 1989.
85. Mason J. A historical view of the stress field. Journal of human stress. 1975;1(2):22.
86. Selye H. A code for coping with stress. AORN Journal. 1977;25(1):35-42.
87. Selye H. Stress and the General Adaptation Syndrome. British Medical Journal. 1950;1(4667):1383-92.
88. Berclaz M. FAIRE AVEC LE STRESS. 2013.
89. Karasek RA. Job Demands, Job Decision Latitude, and Mental Strain: Implications for Job Redesign. Administrative Science Quarterly. 1979;24(2):285-308.
90. De Spiegelaere S, Van Gyes G, De Witte H, Van Hootegem G. Job design, work engagement and innovative work behavior: A multi-level study on Karasek's learning hypothesis. Management Revue. 2015;26(2):123-37.
91. Karasek R, Brisson C, Kawakami N, Houtman I, Bongers P, Amick B. The Job Content Questionnaire (JCQ): an instrument for internationally comparative assessments of psychosocial job characteristics. Journal of occupational health psychology. 1998;3(4):322.
92. Johnson JV, Hall EM. Job strain, work place social support, and cardiovascular disease: a crosssectional study of a random sample of the Swedish working population. American journal of public health. 1988;78(10):1336-42.
93. Siegrist J. Adverse Health Effects of High-Effort/Low-Reward Conditions. Journal of occupational health psychology. 1996;1(1):27-41.
94. Folkman S, Lazarus RS, Gruen RJ, DeLongis A. Appraisal, coping, health status, and psychological symptoms. Journal of personality and social psychology. 1986;50(3):571-9. Epub 1986/03/01.
95. Westman M, Hobfoll SE, Chen S, Davidson OB, Laski S. Organizational stress through the lens of conservation of resources (COR) theory. Exploring interpersonal dynamics: Emerald Group Publishing Limited; 2004. p. 167-220.
96. Hobfoll SE. Social and Psychological Resources and Adaptation. Review of General Psychology. 2002;6(4):307-24.
97. Schaufeli W, Firth-Cozens J, Payne R. Stress in health professionals. Stress in health professionals1999.
98. Delbrouck M. Le burn-out du soignant: le syndrome d'épuisement professionnel: De Boeck Supérieur; 2003.
99. Iacovides A, Fountoulakis K, St Kaprinis GK. The relationship between job stress, burnout and clinical depression. Journal of Affective Disorders. 2003;75:209-21.
100. Leiter MP, Durup J. The discriminant validity of burnout and depression: A confirmatory factor analytic study. Anxiety, Stress, & Coping. 1994;7(4):357-73.
101. Firth H, McIntee J, McKeown P, Britton P. Burnout and professional depression: related

concepts? Journal of Advanced Nursing. 1986;11(6):633-41.
102. Ahola K, Hakanen J. Job strain, burnout, and depressive symptoms: A prospective study among dentists. Journal of Affective Disorders. 2007;104(1):103-10.
103. Melchers MC, Plieger T, Meermann R, Reuter M. Differentiating Burnout from Depression: Personality Matters! Frontiers in Psychiatry. 2015;6:113.
104. Marin C, Carron R. Historical evolution of the concept of somatisation. L'Évolution Psychiatrique. 2002;67(3):506-15.
105. Auxéméry Y. What different clinical entities lie behind the generic terms "somatisation" and "functional disorder"? A cardinal question for therapy. Annales Médico-psychologiques, psychiatric journal. 2014;172(5):400-8.
106. Granger B. [Questionable DSM-5]. La Revue du praticien. 2013;63(4):455-6. Epub 2013/05/21. DSM-5 in question.
107. De Silva P, Hewage C, Fonseka P. Burnout: an emerging occupational health problem. Galle Medical Journal. 2009;14(1).
108. Executive decree no. 94-219 of 14 Safar 1415 corresponding to 23 July 1994 amending and supplementing decree no. 71-215 of 25 August 1971 on the organisation of medical studies.
109. Gautier I. Burn out des médecins De l'Idéal à l'usure. 2004.
110. Galam É. Burnout. L'erreur médicale, le burnout et le soignant: De la seconde victime au premier acteur. Paris: Springer Paris; 2012. p. 123-37.
111. Maslach C, Goldberg J. Prevention of burnout: New perspectives. Applied and preventive psychology. 1998;7(1):63-74.
112. Flajolet A. Flajolet Report, Annex 1, prevention: definitions and comparisons. Ministry of Social Affairs and Health. 2001.
113. Kirouac L. Instruments de mesure et voies thérapeutiques du burn-out: la responsabilité sociale court-circuitée. Reflets: Revue d'intervention sociale et communautaire. 2011;17(1):30-57.
114. Stordeur S, Vandenberghe C, DHoore W. [Predictors of nurses' professional burnout: a study in a university hospital]. Rech Soins Infirm. 1999(59):57-67. Epub 2002/06/01. Predictors of nurses' professional burnout: a study in a university hospital.
115. Tavares MOP. Le burnout chez les soignants facteurs prédisposants et moyens de prévention: Haute Ecole de Santé de Fribourg; 2009.
116. Spickard A, Jr, Gabbe SG, Christensen JF. Mid-career burnout in generalist and specialist physicians. Jama. 2002;288(12):1447-50. Epub 2002/09/24.
117. Blondeau F, Boucher G, Frenette J, Turgeon J. Au sujet des groupes Balint. Canadian Family Physician. 1983;29:1770-1.
118. Lévy A. Analyse des pratiques. Vocabulary of psychosociology. 2016:312-22.
119. Schwartz D. Méthodes statistiques à l'usage des médecins et des biologistes.3ème édition 2003.
120. El Sanharawi M, Naudet F. Understanding logistic regression. Journal français d'ophtalmologie. 2013;36(8):710-5.
121. Guinaud M. Évaluation du burn out chez les internes de médecine générale et étude des facteurs associés 2006.
122. Gallois P, Vallée J-P, Le Noc Y. General practice in crisis: facts and issues. Médecine. 2006;2(5):223-8.
123. Soler JK, Yaman H, Esteva M, Dobbs F, Asenova RS, Katie M, et al. Burnout in European family doctors: the EGPRN study. Family practice. 2008;25(4):245-65.
124. Dyrbye L, Shanafelt T, Balch C, Satele D, Sloan J, Freischlag J. Relationship between workhome conflicts and burnout among American surgeons: a comparison by sex. Archives of surgery (Chicago, Ill: 1960). 2011;146(2):211-7.
125. Galam É. Burn out des médecins libéraux-1re partie: une pathologie de la relation d'aide. Médecine. 2007;3(9):419-21.
126. Galam E, Mouriès R. L'épuisement professionnel des médecins libéraux franciliens: témoignages,

analyses et perspectives. Commission Prévention et santé publique URML íle-de- France June. 2007.
127. Wallace JE, Lemaire JB, Ghali WA. Physician wellness: a missing quality indicator. The Lancet. 2009;374(9702):1714-21.
128. Kalemoglu M, Keskin O. Evaluation of stress factors and burnout in the emergency department staff. Ulusal travma dergisi= Turkish journal of trauma & emergency surgery: TJTES. 2002;8(4):215-9.
129. Hamaideh SH. Burnout, social support, and job satisfaction among Jordanian mental health nurses. Issues Ment Health Nurs. 2011;32(4):234-42.
130. Galam E. Burn out among self-employed doctors Part 3: consequences for the doctor and his patients. Médecine. 2008;4(1): 43-6.
131. Galam É. Burn out des médecins libéraux. Second part: a professional identity called into question. Médecine. 2007;3(10):474-7.
132. Hobbs F. Fear of aggression at work among general practitioners who have suffered a previous episode of aggression. The British journal of general practice : the journal of the Royal College of General Practitioners. 1994;44(386):390-4.
133. Van Dierendonck D, Schaufeli WB, Sixma HJ. Burnout among General Practitioners: A Perspective from Equity Theory. Journal of Social and Clinical Psychology. 1994;13(1):86-100.
134. Laur A. Physicians suffering from burnout. A review of the literature. Medicine. 2014;10(1):34-7.
135. Gaboulaud C. Burnout et addiction au travail chez les médecins généralistes de l'ile de la réunion.Médecine humaine et pathologie. 2016 .<dumas-01364295>.
136. Doghmi N, Massou S, Balkhi H, Haimeur C, Drissi Kamili N. Le burn out, conséquences et solutions : enquête chez les personnels d'anesthésie-réanimation de quatre hôpitaux universitaires marocains. Annales Médico-psychologiques, psychiatric journal. 2013;171(10):700-4.
137. Maranda M-F. La détresse des médecins: un appel au changement: rapport d'enquête de psychodynamique du travail: Presses Université Laval; 2006.
138. The Physicians Foundation. A survey of America's physicians:practice patterns and perspectiveshttp://www.physiciansfoundation.org/healthcare-research/a-survey-of-americasphysicians-practice-patterns-and-perspectives. Accessed October1, 2013.
139. McManus I, Keeling A, Paice E. Stress, burnout and doctors' attitudes to work are determined by personality and learning style: A twelve year longitudinal study of UK medical graduates. BMC Medicine. 2004;2(1):29.
140. Robbe-Kernen M, Kehtari R. Les professionnels de la santé face au burnout. Rev Med Suisse. 2014;443(32):1787-92.
141. Doppia MA, Estryn-Béhar M, Fry C, Guetarni K, Lieutaud T. Comparative survey of burnout syndrome among intensive care anaesthetists and other practitioners in public hospitals in France (SESMAT survey). Annales Françaises d'Anesthésie et de Réanimation. 2011;30(11):782-94.
142. Massou S, Doghmi N, Belhaj A, Aboulaala K, Azendour H, Haimeur C, et al. Survey of burnout syndrome among anaesthesia and intensive care staff in four Moroccan university hospitals. Annales Médico-psychologiques, psychiatric journal. 2013;171(8):538-42.
143. El Kettani A, Serhier Z, Othmani MB, Agoub M, Battas O. Evaluation of the Burnout syndrome in doctors in training at the CHU Ibn Rochd in Casablanca. The Pan African medical journal. 2017;27:243.
144. Oumaya M, Ghanmi L, Baccar Y, Khédira B, Salah KB, Bouzid R. P03-259 Burnout or professional exhaustion syndrome among primary care Tunisian doctors. European Psychiatry: Elsevier; 2009. p. S1258.
145. Maaroufi N, Rzeigui J, Ayari L, Abid Z. Burn-out in emergency care. European Scientific Journal. 2015;11(12).
146. Kacem I, Kalboussi H, Ayoub N, Brahem A, Maoua M, Boughattas W, et al., editors. Burn-out among young doctors: a study conducted in the Sousse region. Annales Médico- psychologiques,

revue psychiatrique; 2017: Elsevier.
147. Guèye M, Moreira PM, Dia DA, Ndiaye-Guèye MD, Kane-Guèye SM, Mbaye M, et al. Le syndrome d'épuisement professionnel chez les étudiants en spécialisation au Centre hospitalier universitaire de Dakar (Sénégal). Annales Médico-psychologiques, psychiatric journal. 2016;174(7):551-6.
148. Dusmesnil H, Serre BS, Régi J-C, Leopold Y, Verger P. Burnout among general practitioners: prevalence and determinants. Santé publique. 2009;21(4):355-64.
149. Bontoux E. Prévalence et facteurs de risque du burnout chez les médecins généralistes du GERS: UNIVERSITÉ TOULOUSE III; 2016.
150. Marcelino G, Cerveira JM, Carvalho I, Costa JA, Lopes M, Calado NE, et al. Burnout levels among Portuguese family doctors: a nationwide survey. BMJ Open. 2012;2(3):e001050.
151. Pedersen AF, Andersen CM, Olesen F, Vedsted P. Risk of Burnout in Danish GPs and Exploration of Factors Associated with Development of Burnout: A Two-Wave Panel Study. International Journal of Family Medicine. 2013;2013:603713.
152. Al-Dubai SAR, Rampal KG. Prevalence and associated factors of burnout among doctors in Yemen. Journal of occupational health. 2010;52(1):58-65. Epub 2009/11/10.
153. Selaihem AA. Prevalence of burnout amongst physicians working in primary care in Riyadh military hospital, Saudi Arabia. 2013.
154. Hussein H, Al Faisal W, Wasfy A, Monsef N, AbdulRahim W, El Sawaf E, et al. Burnout Among Primary Health Care Physicians in Dubai Health Authority Dubai-UAE. Public Health and Preventive Medicine. 2015;1(1):24-7.
155. Elbarazi I, Loney T, Yousef S, Elias A. Prevalence of and factors associated with burnout among health care professionals in Arab countries: a systematic review. BMC Health Services Research. 2017;17(1):491.
156. Carlotto MS, Pizzinato A, Bones Rocha K, de Oliveira-Machado R. Prevalence and factors associated with burnout syndrome in professionals in basic health units. Cienc Trab. 2013;15(47):76-80.
157. Barros Dde S, Tironi MO, Nascimento Sobrinho CL, Neves FS, Bitencourt AG, Almeida Ade M, et al. Intensive care unit physicians: socio-demographic profile, working conditions and factors associated with burnout syndrome. Revista Brasileira de terapia intensiva. 2008;20(3):235-40. Epub 2008/09/01. Plantonistas de unidade de terapia intensiva: perfil socio-demografico, condicoes de trabalho e fatores associados a sindrome de burnout.
158. Shanafelt TD, Boone S, Tan L, Dyrbye LN, Sotile W, Satele D, et al. Burnout and satisfaction with work-life balance among US physicians relative to the general US population. Archives of internal medicine. 2012;172(18):1377-85. Epub 2012/08/23.
159. Vaquin-Villeminey C. Prevalence du Burn out en médecine générale: Enquête nationale auprès de 221 médecins généralistes du réseau sentinelles [Burnout amongst 221 GPs of french sentinel network]: Thesis. Paris: Faculté de médecine René Descartes Paris V; 2007.
160. Bonneterre V, Jolivet A, Lang T, Caroly S, Ehlinger V, Sobaszek A, et al. Evaluation of psychological and organisational constraints (POC) in carers: ORSOSA cohort and applications. Archives des Maladies Professionnelles et de l'Environnement. 2010;71(3):489-92.
161. Taee M, Safizadeh H, Divsalar K. Frequency of burnout among general practitioners of kerman city, 2008. Journal of Kerman University of Medical Sciences. 2010;17(3):268-76.
162. Pereira SM, Fonseca AM, Sofia Carvalho A. Burnout in palliative care: A systematic review. Nursing Ethics. 2011;18(3):317-26.
163. Cooke GP, Doust JA, Steele MC. A survey of resilience, burnout, and tolerance of uncertainty in Australian general practice registrars. BMC Medical Education. 2013;13(1):2.
164. Daloz L, Bénony H. Le sujet en état d'épuisement professionnel: Approche clinique sur une population de soignants. Archives des Maladies Professionnelles et de l'Environnement. 2007;68(2):126-35.

165. Cebrià J, Sobrequés J, Rodríguez C, Segura J. Influence of burnout on pharmaceutical expediture among primary care physicians. Gaceta sanitaria. 2003;17(6):483-9.
166. Al-Shoraian GMJ, Hussain N, Alajmi MF, Kamel MI, El-Shazly MK. Burnout among family and general practitioners. Alexandria Journal of Medicine. 2011;47(4):359-64.
167. Moreira DdS, Magnago RF, Sakae TM, Magajewski FRL. Prevalence of burnout syndrome in nursing staff in a large hospital in south of Brazil. Cadernos de saude publica. 2009;25(7):1559- 68.
168. Abdulghafour YA, Bo-hamra AM, Al-Randi MS, Kamel MI, El-Shazly MK. Burnout syndrome among physicians working in primary health care centers in Kuwait. Alexandria Journal of Medicine. 2011;47(4):351-7.
169. Embriaco N, Azoulay E, Barrau K, Kentish N, Pochard F, Loundou A, et al. High level of burnout in intensivists: prevalence and associated factors. American journal of respiratory and critical care medicine. 2007;175(7):686-92. Epub 2007/01/20.
170. Arigoni F, Bovier PA, Sappino AP. Trend of burnout among Swiss doctors. Swiss medical weekly. 2010;140:w13070. Epub 2010/09/03.
171. Chen K-Y, Yang C-M, Lien C-H, Chiou H-Y, Lin M-R, Chang H-R, et al. Burnout, Job Satisfaction, and Medical Malpractice among Physicians. International Journal of Medical Sciences. 2013;10(11):1471-8.
172. Bagaajav A, Myagmarjav S, Nanjid K, Otgon S, Chae Y. Burnout and job stress among Mongolian doctors and nurses. Industrial health. 2011;49(5):582-8.
173. Amamou B, Bannour AS, Ben Hadj Yahia M, Ben Nasr S, Ben Hadj Ali B. [High prevalence of burnout in the Tunisian units that support terminally ill patients]. The Pan African medical journal. 2014;19:9. Epub 2015/01/15. High prevalence of burnout in the Tunisian units that support terminally ill patients.
174. Sabbah I, Sabbah H, Sabbah S, Akoum H, Droubi N. Burnout among Lebanese nurses: Psychometric properties of the Maslach burnout inventory-human services survey (MBI-HSS). Health. 2012;4(09):644-52.
175. Edwards N, Kornacki MJ, Silversin J. Unhappy doctors: what are the causes and what can be done? BMJ. 2002;324:835-8.
176. CHEMAA F, HADDAD M. Analyse et identification des facteurs de stress professionnel chez les personnels soignants. Le Journal de la Médecine du Travail. 2012; N°17.
177. Peeters MC, Montgomery AJ, Bakker AB, Schaufeli WB. Balancing work and home: How job and home demands are related to burnout. International Journal of Stress Management. 2005;12(1):43.
178. Veyssier-Belot C. Burnout syndrome among physicians. La Revue de medecine interne / founded by the Societe nationale francaise de medecine interne. 2015;36(4):233-6. Epub 2015/01/27. Burnout syndrome among physicians.
179. Aloulou J, Damak R, Masmoudi F, Sidhom O, Amami O. [Burn out in health care providers: a Tunisian study about 142 nurses]. La Tunisie medicale. 2013;91(1):44-9. Epub 2013/02/14. Burn out in health care providers: a Tunisian study about 142 nurses.
180. Torppa MA, Kuikka L, Nevalainen M, Pitkälä KH. Emotionally exhausting factors in general practitioners' work. Scandinavian Journal of Primary Health Care. 2015;33(3):178-83.
181. Suñer-Soler R, Grau-Martín A, Flichtentrei D, Prats M, Braga F, Font-Mayolas S, et al. The consequences of burnout syndrome among healthcare professionals in Spain and Spanish speaking Latin American countries. Burnout Research. 2014;1(2):82-9.
182. Linzer M, Levine R, Meltzer D, Poplau S, Warde C, West CP. 10 bold steps to prevent burnout in general internal medicine. J Gen Intern Med. 2014;29(1):18-20.
183. Kotb AA, Mohamed KA-E, Kamel MH, Ismail MAR, Abdulmajeed AA. Comparison of burnout pattern between hospital physicians and family physicians working in Suez Canal University Hospitals. The Pan African medical journal. 2014;18:164.
184. Hazif-Thomas C, Thomas P. Carer exhaustion and depersonalisation: a motivational trap. NPG Neurology - Psychiatry - Geriatrics. 2011;11(65):188-93.

185. Leiter MP, Frank E, Matheson TJ. Demands, values, and burnout: Relevance for physicians. Canadian Family Physician. 2009;55(12):1224-5.e1-6.
186. Canoui P. Approche de la souffrance des soignants par l'analyse du concept de l'épuisement professionnel, le burn out: considerations psychologiques et éthiques en reanimation pediatrique: PARIS 5, NECKER; 1997.
187. Vela-Bueno A, Moreno-Jiménez B, Rodríguez-Muñoz A, Olavarrieta-Bernardino S, Fernández-Mendoza J, De la Cruz-Troca JJ, et al. Insomnia and sleep quality among primary care physicians with low and high burnout levels. Journal of Psychosomatic Research. 2008;64(4):435-42.
188. Buysse DJ, Reynolds CF, Monk TH, Berman SR, Kupfer DJ. The Pittsburgh Sleep Quality Index: a new instrument for psychiatric practice and research. Psychiatry Research. 1989;28(2):193-213.
189. Blais F, Gendron L, Mimeault V, Morin C. Evaluation of insomnia: validity of 3 questionnaires. L'Encephale. 1997;23(6):447.
190. Shanafelt TD, Balch CM, Bechamps G, Russell T, Dyrbye L, Satele D, et al. Burnout and medical errors among American surgeons. Annals of surgery. 2010;251(6):995-1000. Epub 2009/11/26.
191. Lee FJ, Stewart M, Brown JB. Stress, burnout, and strategies for reducing them: What's the situation among Canadian family physicians? Canadian Family Physician. 2008;54(2):234-5.
192. Alsaqabi FB, Aldousari A, Ismail AE, El-Shazly M. Job satisfaction among physicians in Al-Sabah Hospital, Kuwait. Alexandria Journal of Medicine. 2010;46(2):83-90.
193. Truchot D. Career orientation and burnout in French general practitioners. Psychological reports. 2008;103(3):875-81. Epub 2009/03/27.
194. Popa F, Arafat R, Purcărea VL, Lalà A, Bobirnac G. Occupational Burnout levels in Emergency Medicine-a nationwide study and analysis. Journal of medicine and life. 2010;3(3):207.
195. Kim WO, Moon SJ, Han SS. Contingent Nurses' Burnout and Influencing Factors. Journal of Korean Academy of Nursing. 2010;40(6).
196. Belkhouja K, Elloumi H, Sifaoui K, Romdhane KB, Hamzaoui O, Ayech T, et al. High burnout among resuscitators and emergency physicians: prevalence and risk factors. Réanimation. 2011;20:S149-S52.
197. Ministerial Instruction No. 18 of 27October 2002 on health protection for healthcare workers.

Appendix 1: Executive Decree on the organisation of medical studies

Décret exécutif n° 94-219 du 14 Safar 1415 correspondant au 23 juillet 1994 modifiant et complétant le décret n° 71-215 du 25 août 1971 portant organisation du régime des études médicales.

Le Chef du Gouvernement ;

Sur le rapport du ministre de l'enseignement supérieur et de la recherche scientifique ;

Vu la Constitution, notamment ses articles 81-4 et 116 (alinéa 2) ;

Vu la plate-forme portant consensus national sur la période transitoire ;

Vu la loi n° 85-05 du 16 février 1985 relative à la protection et à la promotion de la santé ;

Vu le décret n° 71-215 du 25 août 1971, modifié, portant organisation du régime des études médicales ;

Vu le décret présidentiel n° 94-92 du 30 Chaoual 1414 correspondant au 11 avril 1994 portant nomination du Chef du Gouvernement ;

Vu le décret présidentiel n° 94-93 du 4 Dhou El Kaada 1414 correspondant au 15 avril 1994 portant nomination des membres du Gouvernement ;

Décrète :

Article. 1er. — Le présent décret a pour objet de modifier et de compléter le décret n° 71-215 du 25 août 1971 portant organisation du régime des études médicales.

Art. 2. — *L'article* 2 du décret n° 71-215 du 25 août 1971 susvisé est modifié comme suit :

"*Art.* 2. — La durée des études en vue du diplôme de docteur en médecine est de sept (7) ans".

Art. 3. — *L'article 4* du décret n° 71-215 du 25 août 1971 susvisé est modifié comme suit :

"*Art.* 4. — Les candidats au diplôme de docteur en médecine doivent être titulaires du diplôme du baccalauréat scientifique, dont les séries sont fixées par le ministre chargé de l'enseignement supérieur, ou d'un titre étranger reconnu équivalent".

Art. 4. — *L'article 5* du décret n° 71-215 du 25 août 1971 susvisé est modifié et complété comme suit :

"*Art. 5.* — Les études en vue du diplôme de docteur en médecine sont divisées en deux cycles et un stage interné.

— Le premier cycle ou cycle pré-clinique comprend les 1ère, 2ème et 3ème années,

— Le second cycle ou cycle clinique comprend, les 4ème, 5ème et 6ème années,

— Le stage interné d'une durée d'une année à plein temps dans les différents services hospitalo-universitaires, en qualité d'interne et le cas échéant au sein de structures de santé publique dont la liste est déterminée par les ministres chargés de l'enseignement supérieur et de la santé".

Art. 5. — *L'article* 6 du décret n° 71-215 du 25 août 1971 susvisé est modifié comme suit :

"*Art. 6.* — Les enseignements pratiques et dirigés composant les deux cycles et le stage interné prévus à l'article 5 ci-dessus, sont obligatoires".

Art. 6. — *L'article 11* du décret n° 71-215 du 25 août 1971 susvisé est modifié comme suit :

"*Art. 11.* — A l'expiration de la septième année et après accomplissement du stage interné, l'étudiant présente un rapport de stage soumis à évaluation d'un comité pédagogique de stage spécialisé, composé d'enseignements de rang magistral".

Art. 7. — *L'article 15* du décret n° 71-215 du 25 août 1971 susvisé est modifié comme suit :

"*Art. 15.* — Les dispositions du présent décret sont applicables à compter de l'année universitaire 1994-1995".

Art. 8. — *L'article* 16 du décret n° 71-215 du 25 août 1971 susvisé est modifié comme suit :

"*Art. 16.* — Un arrêté du ministre chargé de l'enseignement supérieur fixera les conditions d'organisation de la période transitoire applicable aux étudiants en cours de formation".

Art. 9. — Les articles *2, 4, 5, 6, 11, 15* et 16 du décret n° 71-215 du 25 août 1971 susvisé et les dispositions contraires à celles du présent décret sont abrogées.

Art. 10. — Le présent décret sera publié au *Journal officiel* de la République algérienne démocratique et populaire.

Fait à Alger, le 14 Safar 1415 correspondant au 23 juillet 1994.

Mokdad SIFI.

Appendix 2: Geographical and health maps of the wilaya of Sétif

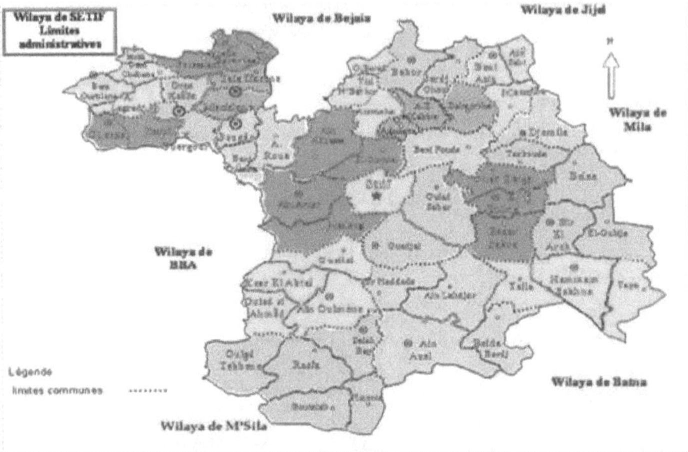

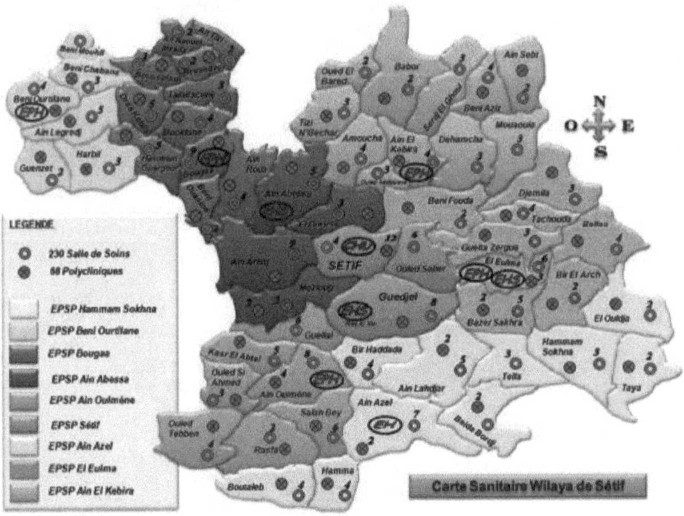

Appendix 3: The questionnaire

Socio-demographic characteristics

Q1- Age : years

Q2- Sex: 1.maleD 2.female

Q3- Marital status: 1.singleQ 2.married□ 3.divorced □ 4.widowed □

Q4- If you are married, is your spouse a doctor? 1.yesQ 2.no □

Q5- How many children are in your care? :

Q6- How many dependents do you have? :

Q7- Do you have any medical condition(s)? 1.yesQ 2.no □

Q8- If yes, which one(s)? :

1.HTAD 2.DiabetesD 3.AsthmaD 4.Thyroid diseaseD 5.Psychiatric condition □ 6.Other s (please specify)

Q9-And for how many years?

1.hypertension....year(s) 2.diabetes...year(s) 3.asthma....year(s) 4.thyroid disease....year(s) 5.psychiatric condition .... year(s) 6.other.years

Characteristics of professional activity

Q10- Location of your practice: 1.EPH □ 2. EPSPQ 3.EH □ 4.EHSQ 5.CHU □

Q11- Do you work in an area: 1. urban □ 2.peri-urbanQ 3.rural □

Q12- Year of graduation :

Q13- Number of years in practice : years

Q14- Do you often have problems getting to work? 1. yes □ 2.no □

Q15- Are you often late for work? 1. yes □ 2.noQ

Q16- How many hours do you work on average per week? hours

Q17- Do you work night shifts? 1.yesD 2.no

Q18- If yes, how many shifts per month?

Q19- Do you think your workload is heavy? 1.yesQ 2.no □

Q20- In your work, are you autonomous in taking decisions? 1 .yesQ 2.no □ Q21- Have you been the victim of aggression (physical or verbal)from patients l.yes □ 2.no □

Q22- If yes, how many times?

Q23-Have you been the victim of aggression (physical or verbal) from their parents? 1.yesD 2.no □

Q24- If yes, how many times?

Q25- Do you feel a sense of injustice towards you in your workplace 1.yesD 2.no □

Q26- If yes, from: 1. generalist colleagues□ 2.specialist colleagues □ 3. paramedical staff □ 4.administration □ 5.other Dcitez

Q27- How would you rate the quality of teamwork? 1. good □ 2.average □ 3. Poor □

Q28- Do you receive support if you need it? 1. yes □ 2.no □

Q29- If yes, from: 1.your colleaguesQ 2.your familyQ 3.your friendsQ 4.others □

Q30- Do you think your salary is satisfactory? 1.yesQ 2.no □

Q31- Have you ever attended any continuing medical education courses? 1. yes Q2.no □

Q32- Do you think this is necessary? 1. yes □ 2.no □

Privacy features

Q33- Do you regularly devote time to activities outside work (cultural activity, sport ...) 1. yes □ 2.no □

Q34- Do you spend enough time with your family? 1. yes □ 2.no □

Q35- Do you have any personal and/or family problems (marital, financial, children's schooling....)? l.yes □ 2.no □

Impact of professional activity

Q36- Do you drink coffee? 1.yesQ 2.no □

Q37- If yes, how many cups/day : cup(s)

Q38- And for how many years? years

Q39- Are you a smoker? 1.yesQ 2.no □

Q40-If yes, number of cigarettes/day : cigarette(s)

Q41- And for how many years? years

Q42- Have you increased your tobacco consumption in the last 12 months?

l.yesH 2.no □

Q43- Do you drink alcohol? 1. yes □ 2.noH

Q44- If yes, for how many years? years

Q45- Do you use drugs? 1.yesH 2.noH

Q46- If yes, for how many years? years

Q47- Have you ever used psychotropic drugs? Louin 2.noH

Q48- If yes, is it? 1. self-medication □ 2.a medical prescription □

Q49- For how many years? years

Q50- How many hours of sleep do you get on average per night? ...hours

Q51- Do you have trouble sleeping? Louin 2.nonH

Q52- In the last 12 months, have you filed one or more work stoppages?

Louin 2.nonH

Q53- If yes, how many? (number of stops)

Q54- Do you have any somatic complaints? 1. yes □ 2.no □

Q55- If yes, which ones (tick)?

Digestive disorders
Headaches
Permanent fatigue
Neurovegetative disorders: palpitations, sweating, hot flushes.
Precordialgia
Musculoskeletal pain
Sleep disorders
Other, please specify

Q56-Are you afraid of committing a medical error? 1. yes □ 2.no □

Q57- If you had to do it all over again, would you study medicine again? 1. yes □ 2.no □

Q58- Do you feel the need to retrain (change jobs)? 1. yes □ 2.no □

Q59- Have you ever had suicidal thoughts? 1. yes □ 2.no □

Q60- Have you heard of burnout syndrome?

1. yes □ 2.no □

Appendix 4: MASLACH BURNOUT INVENTORY (MBI)

MBI Test

Indicate how often you feel what is described in each item:

- Never: 0
- At least a few times a year: 1
- At least once a month: 2
- A few times a month: 3
- Once a week: €4

- A few times a week: 5
- Each day: 6

Item	Frequency						
1. I feel emotionally drained by my work	0	1	2	3	4	5	6
2. I feel exhausted at the end of my working day	0	1	2	3	4	5	6
3. I feel tired when I get up in the morning and have to face another day at work.	0	1	2	3	4	5	6
4. I can easily understand how my patients feel	0	1	2	3	4	5	6
5. I feel that I deal with certain patients in an impersonal way, as if they were objects.	0	1	2	3	4	5	6
6. Working with people all day takes a lot out of me.	0	1	2	3	4	5	6
7. I deal very effectively with the problems of my patients	0	1	2	3	4	5	6
8. I feel I'm cracking up because of my work	0	1	2	3	4	5	6
9. Through my work, I feel I have a positive influence on people.	0	1	2	3	4	5	6
10. I've become more insensitive to people since I got this job	0	1	2	3	4	5	6
11. I'm afraid this job will harden me emotionally	0	1	2	3	4	5	6
12. I feel full of energy	0	1	2	3	4	5	6
13. I feel frustrated by my work	0	1	2	3	4	5	6
14. I feel that I work "too hard" at my job	0	1	2	3	4	5	6
15. I don't really care what happens to some of my patients	0	1	2	3	4	5	6
16. Working in direct contact with people stresses me out too much	0	1	2	3	4	5	6
17. I find it easy to create a relaxed atmosphere with my patients	0	1	2	3	4	5	6
18. I feel rejuvenated when in my work I have been close to my patients.	0	1	2	3	4	5	6
19. I've done a lot of worthwhile things in this job	0	1	2	3	4	5	6
20. I feel at the end of my rope	0	1	2	3	4	5	6
21. In my work, I deal with emotional problems very calmly	0	1	2	3	4	5	6
22. I have the impression that my patients blame me for some of their problems	0	1	2	3	4	5	6

Breakdown of the 22 items

Burnout: questions 1.2.3.6.8.13.14.16.20.

Depersonalisation: questions 5.10.11.15.22.

Personal achievement: questions 4.7.9.12.17.18.19.21.

For each dimension, the responses to the items that make it up are added together to obtain scores.

MBI French scale

	MBI dimensions - French version		
Burnout score	EE	DP	AP
High	> 30	> 12	< 33
Moderate	18 - 29	6 - 11	34 - 39
Low	< 17	< 5	> 40

MBI (Fontaine translation) [15]

- The level of emotional exhaustion is considered low, moderate or high for scores respectively set at < 17, 18-29, > *30.*
- For the degree of depersonalisation, the scores are respectively set at < 5, 6-11, > 12.
- For personal fulfilment, the scores are respectively set at < 33, 34-39, > 40 [3].

The personal fulfilment dimension is **inversely** related to the other two MBI dimensions: a low personal fulfilment score indicates a high level of burnout.

The absence (or low level) of burnout can be assessed through low scores on the emotional exhaustion and depersonalisation scales, combined with a high score for personal fulfilment.

A high score on the EE dimension **or** the PD dimension **or** a low score on the PA dimension is sufficient to speak of burnout.

Annex 5: MINISTERIAL INSTRUCTION No. 18 OF 27 OCTOBER 2002 ON HEALTH PROTECTION FOR HEALTH CARE STAFF

PEOPLE'S DEMOCRATIC REPUBLIC OF ALGERIA
MINISTERE DE LA SANTE DE LA POPULATION
ET DE LA REFORME HOSPITALIERE

THE MINISTER
ADDRESSEES :

- Dear Health and Population Directors.

For communication to the Health Sector Directors.

- The Chief Executive Officers of the University Hospitals.
- The Directors of the Etablissements Hospitaliers Spécialisés.

Healthcare staff of all categories, and particularly nursing staff, who are in contact with patients, especially in emergency units and wards, intensive care units and those dealing with serious pathologies, are often faced with extreme situations in their constant battle against the suffering and illness of the patients in their care.

They may be subject to significant physical constraints at work, but also to increasing mental constraints in busy departments, as a result of problems caused by organisational and relational constraints, or relating to their experience of their work, which may combine dissatisfaction, lack of participation in decision-making and even feelings of insecurity and danger at work.

All these constraints can lead to psychological suffering among care staff when working conditions are unfavourable, and can lead to stress at work, the extreme manifestation of which is burn-out syndrome.

The generic term "psychosocial risks" is used to describe all these constraints, and it is important to be aware of their potential impact on the deteriorating health of healthcare workers.

These risks need to be prevented in the same way as the physical, chemical and biological risks to which healthcare workers may be exposed, depending on their workstation.

In order to better assess all the risks, including psychosocial risks, in the various health establishments, to prevent their effects and to provide early care for health workers in stressful situations, a preventive approach should be implemented as soon as possible in all establishments, based on the analysis of activities and working conditions, and on medico-environmental monitoring in the care environment.

The solutions to the problems identified can then be considered at both individual and collective/organisational level.

Such a preventive approach must be initiated and sponsored by the management and consultative bodies of the establishments, in liaison with the workers' representatives, in order to bring together the conditions necessary for its success. It must also be supported by the establishments' occupational medicine departments and the health and safety committees, which were the subject of instruction no. 10 of 6 May 2002 concerning their establishment.

This approach must be part of efforts to improve the quality of care and must be regularly evaluated.

Occupational health services must therefore focus their activities more on risk assessment and prevention by :

1. Carrying out regular and sustained analysis of workstations, activities and working conditions in all departments and care units, paying particular attention to the mental workload, taking into account all parameters, i.e. the organisation of working time, constraints on the pace of work, autonomy and scope for initiative, the work group and contact with patients and the public.
2. Assessing psychopathological effects.
3. Issuing the appropriate fitness notices, taking into account both the physical and psychological constraints of the workstations, depending on the abilities of the health care staff concerned, prior to any new recruitment or new assignment and at the time of the periodic medical check-ups or return medical check-ups provided for in the regulations relating to occupational medicine.
4. Proposing any adjustments to workstations required to protect the physical and mental health of

staff, taking into account the need to ensure the availability and continuity of care.

5. Proposing the necessary transfers when the adaptation of workstations is not compatible with the normal operation of the department.

6. Suggesting to management and the heads of the departments concerned changes and improvements to be made to the running of departments and care units when major malfunctions are noted and are likely to deteriorate the state of health of staff.

The Health and Safety Committees must operate regularly and take on board the opinions and recommendations of the occupational physicians, in liaison with the heads of department concerned, with a view to constantly improving the working conditions of hospital staff.

They should be the main forum in which staff grievances about their working conditions and proposals from occupational health services can be addressed in terms of collective prevention of physical, biological and chemical risks, as well as those linked to organisational and relational constraints.

Each health care establishment must therefore draw up an activity plan for the protection of workers' health, with deadlines and indicators for the various actions taken to improve the working conditions of health care staff.

The business plan must involve both management and employee representatives.

The implementation of business plans and the extent to which they have been put into practice will play an important role in the assessment of healthcare establishments.

I would like to place particular emphasis on the implementation of this system and its optimal operation, which requires special attention from the Boards of Directors, Management Boards and Scientific and Medical Councils of health establishments.

A report on its implementation must be drawn up by December 2002.

The Minister for Health, Population and Hospital Reform

SUMMARY

متلازمة الإرهاق المهني أو الإحتراق النفسي

دراسة وصفيّة عند الأطبّاء العامّون في ولاية سطيف

ملخص

تعدُّ متلازمة الإرهاق المهني أو الإحتراق النّفسي (**Burnout**) أو ما يعرف اختصارا بـ (**BO**) عند الأطبّاء العامّون مشكلة حقيقية في الصّحة العمومية. رغم ذلك، فإنَ الدّراسات المنشورة حوله قليلة. ويعرف بـ: "الإجهاد أو الإرهاق العاطفي (**EE**) ، ومتلازمة تبدد الشخصية (**DP**) ، ومحدودية تحقيق الذّات (**AP**) حيث تظهر أعراضها عند الأشخاص الذين لديهم علاقات مهنيّة مع الآخرين". تهدف هذه الدّراسة إلى تقييم مدى انتشار هذه المتلازمة و أبعادها الثّلاثة عندهذه الفئة . تمّ إجراء مسح وصفي عرضي على عيّنة تمثيلية من **463** طبيب عام يمارسون في المرافق الصحية ومستشفيات ولاية سطيف خلال الفترة الممتدة من ديسمبر **2016** إلى ديسمبر **2017**. وجاء معدّل انتشار الاحتراق بـ **49**٪ والاحتراق الشديد بنسبة **3.2**٪، حيث سجّل الأطباء العامّون إرهاقا عاطفيا بنسبة **37.8**٪ من الحالات، كما أن نسبة تبدد الشخصية المرتفع (**DP**) جاءت بنسبة **12.3**٪ وجاءت محدودية تحقيق الذات المنخفضة (**AP**) عند **17.7**٪ من الحالات. وارتبطت الأبعاد الثلاثة للاحتراق بالعديد من العوامل عند الأطباء العامين، غير أن عبء العمل يبدو أنه من الأخطار الرئيسية ، وتتضح عواقبه من خلال الجسدنة أو الشكاوى الجسدية، والخوف من ارتكاب أي خطأ طبي، واستهلاك المؤثرات العقلية، وكذلك في الرغبة في تغيير الوظيفة. لهذا الغرض، يتعين إدراك إمكانية التأثير المباشر لهذا العرض على تدهور الحالة الصحية للأطباء العامين. لذلك نرى أنه من الضروري انتهاج أسلوب وقائي يركز على تحليل ظروف العمل والترصد الطبي والبيئي في الوسط العلاجي، مع ضرورة إشراك وإقحام خدمات طب العمل الذي يبدو حتمية في هذه الحالة.

الكلمات الدالة : - الإرهاق المهني - الإحتراق النفسي- الإرهاق العاطفي - تبدد الشخصية - تحقيق الذات - أطباء عامون.

BURNOUT SYNDROME: DESCRIPTIVE STUDY OF GENERAL PRACTITIONERS IN THE WILAYA OF SETIF

SUMMARY

Burnout syndrome in general practitioners (GPs) is a real public health issue. Few studies have been published on the subject in our country. It is "a syndrome of emotional exhaustion (EE), depersonalisation (DP) and reduced personal accomplishment (AP) that appears in individuals who are professionally involved with others". The aim of this study was to assess the prevalence of this syndrome and its three dimensions among GPs. A descriptive cross-sectional survey was conducted on a representative sample of 463 GPs practising in health and hospital facilities in the wilaya of Sétif during the period from December 2016 to December 2017. The prevalence of BO was 49% with 3.2% of severe BO. GPs were in high EE in 37.8%, PD was high in 12.3% and PA was low in 17.7%. Several factors were associated with the three dimensions of OOP, but workload appeared to be the major risk. The consequences of OO appear to be somatic complaints, fear of committing a medical error, use of psychotropic drugs and the desire to change profession. To this end, it is imperative to be aware of the possible impact of OB on the deterioration of GPs' state of health. A preventive approach centred on the analysis of working conditions and on medical and environmental surveillance in the care environment is essential. The support and involvement of occupational medicine departments would appear to be a matter of course.

Keywords : Burnout (BO) - Emotional exhaustion (EE) - Depersonalisation (DP) - Personal fulfilment (PA) - General practitioners (GP)

FSC
www.fsc.org
MIX
Papier | Fördert gute Waldnutzung
FSC® C083411

Kolibri 360 GmbH
Ferdinand-Jühlke-Straße 7
99095 Erfurt, Deutschland
produktsicherheit@kolibri360.de

Druck:
CPI Druckdienstleistungen GmbH
im Auftrag der
Kolibri 360 GmbH
Ferdinand-Jühlke-Str. 7
99095 Erfurt